Series in Psychopathology

Series Editor
Lauren B. Alloy

Michael W. O'Hara

Postpartum Depression

Causes and Consequences

With a Foreword by Lee S. Cohen, M.D.

With 22 Illustrations

Springer-Verlag
New York Berlin Heidelberg London Paris
Tokyo Hong Kong Barcelona Budapest

Michael W. O'Hara, Ph.D.
Department of Psychology
The University of Iowa
Iowa City, IA 52242-1407

Library of Congress Cataloging-in-Publication Data
O'Hara, Michael W.
Postpartum depression: causes and consequences/Michael W. O'Hara.
p. cm.
Includes bibliographical references and index.
ISBN 0-387-94261-0. — ISBN 3-540-94261-0
1. Postpartum depression. I. Title.
[DNLM: 1. Depression—etiology. 2. Puerperal Disorders—psychology. 3. Psychotic Disorders. 4. Pregnancy—psychology. 5. Depressive Disorder—therapy. WM 171 O36p 1994]
RG852.O33 1994
618.7'6—dc20 94-7180

Printed on acid-free paper.

Production coordinated by Chernow Editorial Services, Inc., and managed by Francine McNeill; manufacturing supervised by Jacqui Ashri.
Typeset by Best-set Typesetter Ltd., Hong Kong

9 8 7 6 5 4 3 2 1

ISBN-13: 978-1-4613-8418-2 e-ISBN-13: 978-1-4613-8416-8
DOI: 10.1007/978-1-4613-8416-8

To Jane, Jeffrey, and Andrew for their love
and support
and to my parents, Bill and Colleen

Foreword

What is the prevalence of mood disorders during pregnancy and the postpartum period; does the prevalence vary compared to nonchildbearing women? What are the psychosocial and neurobiologic factors that predict risk for postpartum mood disorders? *Postpartum Depression: Causes and Consequences* by Michael W. O'Hara synthesizes a series of efforts to address these and other difficult questions. It is a clear, cohesive, and carefully prepared work, which serves not only as a review of more than a decade of research, but also as a charge for future investigation regarding unanswered questions about postpartum mood disturbance.

Depression after childbirth is one of the most prevalent complications in modern obstetrics. Nonetheless, the subject of postpartum mood disorders remains understudied. Some investigators pursue nosologic debates regarding the extent to which postpartum depression should be considered a discreet diagnostic entity. Others have tried to identify biologic or psychosocial factors that are uniquely associated with puerperal illness. More recent efforts have begun to focus on the need to identify predictors of risk for developing depression during pregnancy and the postpartum period. Identification of women "at risk" can lead to prophylactic treatment strategies that attenuate such risk, thereby limiting morbidity associated with untreated depression and the impact of maternal psychiatric disorder on child development.

The current volume is an elegant review not only of the work performed by Michael W. O'Hara and his colleagues at the University of Iowa, but also of the dozens of investigations designed to answer questions regarding the causes and sequalae of postpartum mood disturbance. The book is greater than the sum of its parts. On the one hand, it is about the relationship between childbirth and mood disorders. On another level, it is about replacing myths regarding pregnancy and the puerperium. This is achieved by subjecting difficult questions to rigorous and systematic investigation. The book outlines the methodologic and conceptual framework from which a number of scientific investigations have been derived in an effort to integrate more clearly the factors that potentially contribute to postpartum mood disturbance.

The scope of research reviewed in the text is vast. Findings of similar rates of mood disorder in childbearing and nonchildbearing women are reviewed, and the implications are discussed. Pregnancy and the puerperium may not impact on the natural course of mood disorder, and thus, the postpartum period does not appear to be a period of particular risk for the development of nonpsychotic major depression. What does appear to place women at risk for postpartum depression, however, is a personal or family history of depression. This finding, which is noted in several of the studies discussed in the book, has extraordinary implications given the prevalence of mood disorder in women during their childbearing years and the extent to which these populations of women "at risk" frequently go unidentified. The absence of conclusive findings of specific neuroendocrine dysregulation associated with puerperal illness or psychosocial variables that uniformly correlate with postpartum depression combined with the predictive value of such variables as personal or family history of depression ultimately lead the reader to conclude that mood disturbance during childbearing is indeed a complicated affair. It is conceivably a phenomenon derived from a convergence of biologic and psychosocial factors that interact with preexisting vulnerability.

Perhaps the most compelling aspect of *Postpartum Depression: Causes and Consequences* is found not in a single table or statistical analysis, but rather in the implied mandate that springs from the studies described—namely, to screen for so prevalent a disorder (and for factors that may predict its emergence) in such nonresearch settings as primary-care medicine and obstetrics and gynecology. If personal and family history of mood disorder as well as past history of postpartum depression appears to be strongly associated with depression during pregnancy and the puerperium, then there is a clear need to screen for mood disorder in settings in which women seek medical treatment. Screening of women at potential risk for mood disturbance during pregnancy and the postpartum period is the first step toward identification of these women and toward providing closer follow-up and early intervention, if necessary. Our ability to predict particular vulnerability to the onset of mood disturbance during pregnancy or the puerperium also opens the door to the possibility of studying prophylactic strategies to attenuate such risk.

Appropriate screening before, during, and after pregnancy may help identify women with mood disturbances responsive to a wide spectrum of therapies. Identification of greater numbers of women with postpartum psychiatric illness must be complemented by intensive efforts to treat these women. Risks of untreated mood disorder including chronic affective disorder are well described. Of equal concern is the evolving evidence suggesting an adverse impact of maternal mood disorder on child development. If the current text helps legitimize puerperal illness, then our next task is to insist on its treatment. To that end, this volume clearly helps pave the way.

Lee S. Cohen, M.D.
Boston, Massachusetts

Acknowledgments

The research described in this volume was supported by National Institute of Mental Health Grant MH39383 to Michael W. O'Hara. The writing of this volume was supported by the University of Iowa Faculty Scholar program. Many colleagues and students collaborated on this research and made significant contributions to it, including Ellen Zekoski, Laurie Philipps, Ellen Wright, Michael Varner, Janet Schlechte, and David Lewis. Expert consultation for various aspects of this research was provided by Daniel Russell, Jon Lemke, Don Routh, and Linda Whitaker. I also thank Mary Walling for her critical reading of an earlier version of this volume. Finally, I wish to thank all of the women who so generously gave of themselves and their time. This work would not have been possible without them.

Michael W. O'Hara
Iowa City, Iowa

Contents

1
Introduction

The prospect of having a baby is met with eager anticipation by most women and families. Children bring great joy to the lives of families and often represent a major source of life fulfillment for women. Unfortunately, for some women the postpartum period is a time of great difficulty and emotional distress. An emotional disturbance, often depression, may significantly reduce the pleasure a woman experiences in mothering; it may even interfere with the development of a positive mother-child relationship. Such emotional disturbances may be long-standing in the individual, or they may develop suddenly after delivery. They may be mild and brief in duration, or they may be severe and persist for months or years. As a group, these emotional disturbances have often been called *postpartum depression*. However, it has been common to divide emotional disturbances in the postpartum period into three groups that are differentiated largely on the basis of severity: (1) postpartum blues, (2) postpartum depression, and (3) postpartum psychosis.

This volume will be primarily concerned with postpartum depression and, to a lesser extent, postpartum blues. Postpartum depression has been a major focus of our research for the past 15 years at the University of Pittsburgh and the University of Iowa. During this time research on postpartum depression has burgeoned in both the United States and Europe. We have conducted three major prospective studies of postpartum depression, the first two of which will be summarized in the next chapter. The rest of this monograph will present the results of our most recent study on the psychological, social, and hormonal factors in postpartum depression and postpartum blues.

The purpose of this chapter is to provide a background for the material that is to follow. The importance of the study of postpartum depression will be addressed first. Postpartum blues and postpartum depression will be described next. Finally, information regarding their epidemiology, etiology, and treatment will be presented.

Why Study Postpartum Mood Disorders?

In 1992 there were about 4,084,000 live births in the United States. Roughly 40% of these births were complicated by a mild mood disturbance, the *postpartum blues* (in this volume, often called the blues). More importantly, approximately 10% of all women experienced a major depression after delivery, and 0.2% of all women became psychotic after delivery. These percentages add up to a great deal of suffering each year by women and their families. Although mood disorders are relatively common (Myers et al., 1984), particularly among women, the difficulty of coping simultaneously with a mood disturbance and a new baby can be overwhelming. Moreover, maternal depression that is present during the postpartum period may presage continuing problems with depression (Philipps & O'Hara, 1991). Also, maternal depression and associated problems such as marital distress appear to have negative implications for the adjustment of children of all ages (Downey & Coyne, 1990).

Childbirth is a life event that by almost any standard is stressful (Holmes & Rahe, 1967). As a life event, childbirth may be better labeled *childbearing,* a process that begins at conception and continues until some months after delivery. That is, even while childbirth (the delivery of the child) is a rather discrete event, what is important physically, psychologically, and socially encompasses much more than the delivery itself. The complexity of childbearing as a life event offers the researcher interested in the relation between stress and depression a rich and important context in which to test hypotheses regarding potential biological, psychological, and social causal factors in depression. Much of the recent North American research on postpartum depression, particularly done by psychologists, has been in the service of testing psychological models of depression (Cutrona, 1983; Manly, McMahon, Bradley, & Davidson, 1982; O'Hara, Rehm, & Campbell, 1982; O'Hara, Schlechte, Lewis, & Varner, 1991).

The lay public also has become increasingly concerned about postpartum mood disorders. National organizations such as Postpartum Support International and Depression After Delivery have emerged as support and advocacy groups for women who have experienced psychological distress after delivery. These groups are also interested in education and the development of knowledge about postpartum disorders, particularly in the areas of treatment and prevention. As a consequence, their members exert pressure on the mental health community to apply resources toward increasing services for women with postpartum mood disorders. Related to this phenomenon have been recent self-help books for postpartum-depressed women such as *The New Mother Syndrome: Coping with Postpartum Stress and Depression* (Dix, 1985).

The answers to the question posed at the beginning of this section—that is, Why study postpartum mood disorders?—should be apparent. To summarize these answers, problems of poor maternal adjustment during the postpartum period have important negative implications for both the new mother and her family. Additionally, there is a scientific interest in testing models of depression in the context of childbearing. Finally, childbearing women are demanding answers to their questions about the causes and consequences of and the treatments for postpartum depression.

The Range of Postpartum Mood Disorders

This volume will be primarily concerned with postpartum depression and postpartum blues; however, before reviewing this literature, a brief discussion of postpartum psychosis is in order. *Postpartum psychosis* is the most severe form of psychiatric disturbance in the puerperium (i.e., the first 6 to 12 weeks after delivery) and it complicates about 2 in 1,000 deliveries. Women experiencing postpartum psychosis are grossly impaired in their ability to function, usually because of hallucinations or delusions. In other cases women may be disturbed by severely depressed mood or confusion. Many of these women suffer from affective disorder; however, schizophrenia is not an uncommon diagnosis for a postpartum psychosis (see Case History 1.1). Although the DSM-II (American Psychiatric Association [APA], 1968) did contain a category "294.4 Psychosis with childbirth" (p. 31), postpartum psychosis (and the blues and depression) are nowhere listed in the DSM-III-R (APA, 1987) or ICD-9 (World Health Organization [WHO], 1978), nor is postpartum psychosis listed in DSM-IV or ICD-10. It is generally believed that there are not enough unique features of postpartum psychosis or other disorders to warrant separate diagnostic categories (Purdy & Frank, 1993).

One important feature of postpartum psychosis is that it tends to occur in close proximity to childbirth. In fact, the first 30 days postpartum represent a very high-risk period for the onset of a new episode of psychosis (Kendell, Chalmers, & Platz, 1987; McNeil, 1986; Nott, 1982). Figure 1.1 illustrates this phenomenon graphically. Kendell et al. (1987) linked obstetric and psychiatric records for more than 50,000 women over a 20-year period in Edinburgh, Scotland. They plotted the number of psychiatric admissions for psychosis for a period spanning 2 years prior to delivery to 2 years subsequent to delivery (a total span of 4 years) for every subject and found that the vast majority of psychiatric admissions for psychosis occurred in the first 90 days after delivery. For example, they determined that the risk of hospitalization for psychosis within 30 days of delivery was 22 times greater than the risk of being hospitalized for psychosis during a 30-day nonchildbearing period. These findings make clear that the postpartum period is a high-risk time for psychosis in childbearing women. The extent to which the postpartum period is also a high-risk time for nonpsychotic postpartum depression was one of the

Case History 1.1. Postpartum psychosis: Paranoid schizophrenia

Mrs. Hines, a 28-year-old schoolteacher, was admitted to the hospital $2\frac{1}{2}$ weeks following cesarean delivery of her first child. At the time of her admission, she had not eaten or slept for 2 days. She had the delusional belief that her brother-in-law was really the father of her baby. Two previous pregnancies had ended at 6 months' gestation due to an incompetent cervix. Mrs. Hines had severe reactions to these miscarriages but did not seek treatment. She had no personal or family history of psychiatric illness. Two days prior to hospitalization, Mrs. Hines complained that there was "something wrong" with her son's penis, at which point she threatened him with a pair of scissors and began verbally to attack relatives. She presented to the hospital with flat affect, although she was well oriented and her memory was intact. While hospitalized Mrs. Hines was very suspicious and believed that her thoughts and words were being recorded and used against her. She was diagnosed as having paranoid schizophrenia and received 20 electroconvulsive treatments, as well as therapy with chlorpromazine for 10 days. She was discharged after $2\frac{1}{2}$ months, still somewhat paranoid. At follow-up 6 weeks later, she evidenced no looseness of associations, inappropriate affect, or paranoid ideation. Mrs. Hines remained well for 13 years, when she relapsed and was rehospitalized.

Note: Case History 1.1 is from "Postpartum mood disorders—Detection and prevention" by M.W. O'Hara & J. Engeldinger, 1989, *The Female Patient, 14,* p. 25. Copyright 1989 by Core Publishing. Reprinted by permission.

major questions addressed in the study that will be described in this volume.

Postpartum depression and the blues are much less severe than postpartum psychosis and much more common. Although there are clear differences in the severity of the typical cases of these disorders (psychosis, depression, blues), it is unclear whether they actually represent three different disorders. It has been proposed that postpartum mood disorders range along a continuum of severity, from little or no disturbance to severe disturbance (O'Hara & Zekoski, 1988). There are no natural dividing points to separate one of these disorders from the other, and women at the boundaries will be very similar to each other. Nevertheless, the rest of this review will be limited to studies of nonpsychotic disorders that encompass mainly depression and the blues. The interested reader is

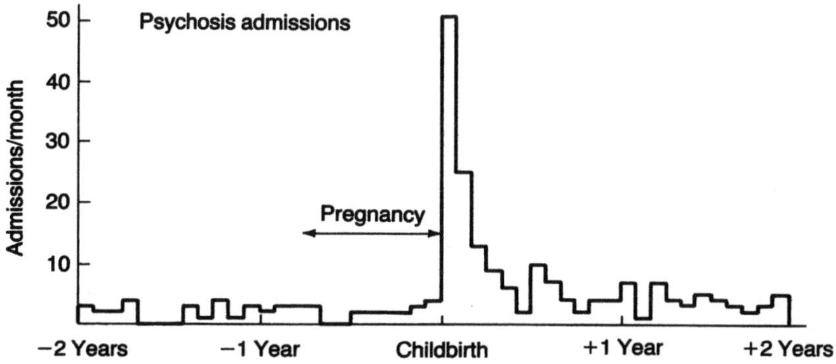

FIGURE 1.1. Risk for hospitalization for psychosis associated with childbirth. From "Epidemiology of puerperal psychoses" by R. Kendell, J. Chalmers, & C. Platz, 1987, *British Journal of Psychiatry, 150,* 662–673. Copyright 1987 by the Royal College of Psychiatrists. Reprinted by permission of the publisher.

directed to other comprehensive reviews of the postpartum psychosis literature (Hamilton & Harberger, 1992; Kendell, 1985).

Description and Diagnosis

Blues

Mild dysphoria during the first week after delivery is a common experience for childbearing women (O'Hara, 1991; Stein, 1982). Symptoms such as depressed mood, crying spells, irritability, anxiety, mood lability, confusion, and sleep and appetite disturbance are often reported (Hamilton, 1962; Kennerley & Gath, 1989a; Pitt, 1973; Stein, 1982). Despite the connotation of the "blues," sadness and depression are not usually the most common symptoms. Crying, confusion, anxiety, and mood lability are often much more prominent (Kennerley & Gath, 1989a). Typically, symptoms begin within a few days of delivery and may last anywhere from a few hours to several days. Frequency or severity of blues symptoms generally peaks between the third and fifth postpartum days (Iles, Gath, & Kennerley, 1989; Kendell, McGuire, Connor, & Cox, 1981; Kennerley & Gath, 1989a). Table 1.1 presents a list of 28 symptoms found by Kennerley and Gath to be common after delivery and to peak on about postpartum day 5.

A variety of criteria have been used to diagnose the blues. For example, Pitt (1973) identified women as having the blues if they "felt tearful and depressed in the puerperium" (defined as within the first week to 10 days after delivery). Yalom, Lunde, Moos, and Hamburg (1968) employed a similar procedure. Probably the best validated of the blues measures is

TABLE 1.1. Symptoms of the postpartum blues.

1. Tearful	15. Emotionally numb, without feelings
2. Mentally tense	16. Depressed
3. Able to concentrate	17. Overemotional
4. Low-spirited	18. Happy
5. Elated	19. Confident
6. Helpless	20. Changeable in your spirits
7. Finding it difficult to show your feelings	21. Tired
8. Alert	22. Irritable
9. Forgetful, muddled	23. Crying without being able to stop
10. Anxious	24. Lively
11. Wishing you were alone	25. Oversensitive
12. Mentally relaxed	26. Up and down in your mood
13. Brooding on things	27. Restless
14. Feeling sorry for yourself	28. Calm, tranquil

Note: For the positive symptoms (e.g., 5, 8, 12), it is their absence that reflects a symptom of the blues (from "Maternity Blues I: Detection and measurement by questionnaire" by H. Kennerley & D. Gath, 1989, *British Journal of Psychiatry, 155,* 356–362).

the Blues Questionnaire (Kennerley & Gath, 1989a), which was developed to assess the frequency of the 28 blues symptoms listed in Table 1.1. The Blues Questionnaire was also used to classify women as having or not having the blues during the first 10 days postpartum. Women whose total blues score on any one day was greater than the mean *peak* blues scores for the whole group of women (i.e., all women in the sample) were classified as having the blues. Other methods of classification have included using a predetermined cutoff on a self-report measure of blues symptoms (Stein, 1980) and using cutoffs from several self-report measures of blues-related symptoms (Handley, Dunn, Waldron, & Baker, 1980). Our own blues measures were based on the earlier work of several investigators (Handley et al., 1980; Kendell et al., 1981). Our work in this area is described more fully in chapters 3, 4, and 7. Case History 1.2 illustrates many of the common characteristics of the postpartum blues.

Depression

Interest in depression after childbirth is of a more recent origin than interest in the blues and psychosis (O'Hara, 1991). It was not until Pitt (1968) described what he termed "atypical" depression following childbirth that attention began to be focused on those depressions that were less serious than the typical postpartum psychosis. Unlike the blues or psychosis, major (or minor) postpartum depressions do not necessarily begin soon after delivery (O'Hara & Zekoski, 1988). For some women postpartum depression will have carried over from pregnancy, while for other women a depressive episode may not begin until several months after

Case History 1.2. Postpartum blues

Mrs. Smith was a 24-year-old woman, married for about 4 years, who was employed full time as a medical technologist. The pregnancy, her first, was planned, and Mrs. Smith and her husband actively prepared for childbirth. Mrs. Smith had experienced a major depression about $4\frac{1}{2}$ years prior to her pregnancy. Both of her parents and her two sisters had experienced major depression or dysthymia during their lifetimes. After a relatively brief labor and a vaginal delivery, Mrs. Smith delivered a full-term boy. The only medical problem noted at the delivery was the possibility that the baby had an inguinal hernia.

Mrs. Smith felt well for the first 3 days postpartum; her mood was generally positive. By day 4 postpartum, she reported feeling increasingly depressed, tearful, anxious, panicky, and tired. These experiences persisted for about 10 days. She noted that around 7:00 P.M. each evening she would become very tearful and her mood would be at the lowest for the day. She felt that she could not control her crying. Worry about her son was another significant problem for her. She was concerned about whether his behaviors were normal or not, about his eating, and she felt uptight when other people held her son. She also noted that she was very irritable and took much of her anger out on her husband. In retrospect she later said that she had too much company and they stayed too long. The major problems that she identified during the first 2 weeks postpartum were some negative experiences with the hospital staff, lack of support from her spouse, being overwhelmed by the demands of infant care, problems feeding the baby, and having a very disorganized house. By 2 weeks postpartum, Mrs. Smith began to feel better and experienced no further dysphoric mood during the postpartum period.

delivery. Figure 1.2, adapted from Watson, Elliott, Rugg, and Brough (1984), illustrates the diversity of onsets and durations of postpartum depression.

Recent studies of postpartum depression have used traditional diagnostic criteria (e.g., Research Diagnostic Criteria, or RDC [Spitzer, Endicott, & Robins, 1978], DSM-III [APA, 1980], or ICD-9 [WHO, 1978]) to define these depressions. Major symptoms include dysphoric mood, loss of interest in usually pleasurable activities, change in appetite, change in sleep, fatigue, excessive or reduced motor behavior, guilt or self-deprecation, difficulties in concentrating or making decisions, and suicidal thoughts. These symptoms are the ones used to make a diagnosis of major depressive episode using DSM-III-R criteria (APA, 1987). Table 1.2 presents the RDC (Spitzer et al., 1978) major and minor depression

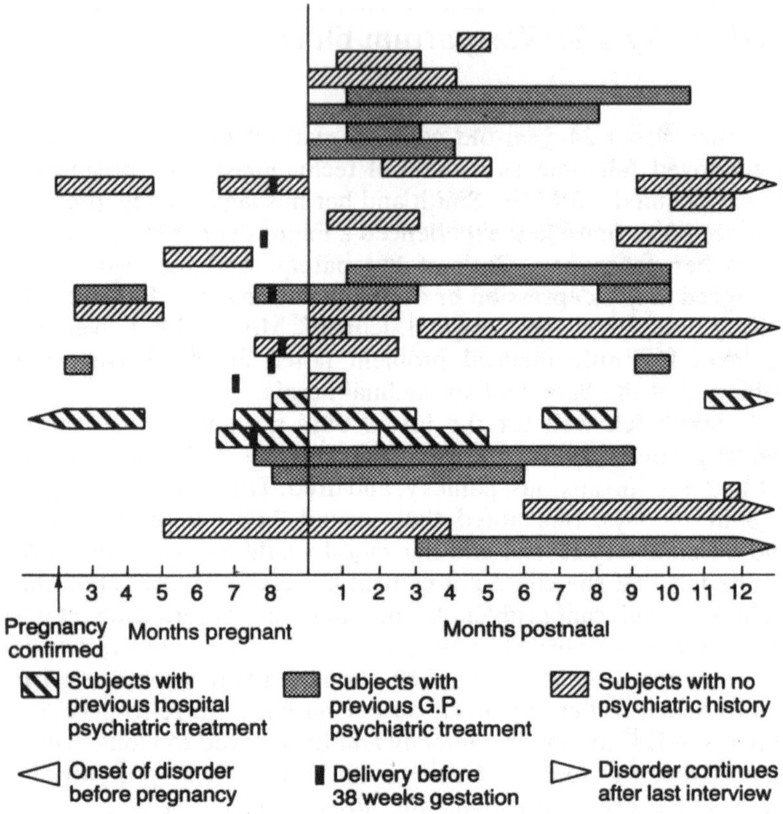

FIGURE 1.2. Onset and duration of depressions beginning during pregnancy and after delivery. From "Psychiatric disorder in pregnancy and the first postnatal year" by J. Watson, S. Elliott, A. Rugg, & D. Brough, 1984, *British Journal of Psychiatry, 144,* 453–462. Copyright 1984 by the Royal College of Psychiatrists. Adapted by permission of the publisher.

TABLE 1.2. Symptoms of major and minor depression (based on research diagnostic criteria).

Major depression symptoms	Minor depression symptoms
Appetite disturbance	Excessive pessimism
Sleep disturbance	Feelings of inadequacy
Excessive fatigue	Irritability
Loss of interest in pleasurable activities	Demandingness or dependency
Excessive guilt	Self-pity
Difficulties in thinking and concentration	Excessive somatic concerns
Thoughts of suicide	Tearfulness or sad face
Psychomotor disturbance	Brooding about unpleasant events

Case History 1.3. Postpartum depression

Mrs. Jones was 26 years old, married, and experiencing her first pregnancy. She had a college degree and was working full-time as a pharmacist. Her husband was 36 years old and in school. Mrs. Jones was the oldest of three siblings; her parents were both still living but had separated about 4 years before her pregnancy. Mr. and Mrs. Jones were actively preparing for childbirth. The pregnancy was planned and Mrs. Jones and her husband were happy about it. She did report some negative feelings, however, about her upcoming experience with childbirth.

The initial interview with Mrs. Jones took place in January. Mrs. Jones reported having felt irritable since the previous October. She had few other symptoms; however, she did find that some aspects of her work and relationships with her family were mildly impaired. She reported a previous episode of depression about 5 years earlier when she was a college student. It lasted about 5 months, and she was seen at the university counseling center for treatment. She reported that she had had many previous similar episodes (6). However, there was no evidence of any other psychiatric difficulty in her history.

Mrs. Jones said that her mother had experienced recurrent unipolar depressions at least once a year over many years, beginning at age 33. Her father had a long history of alcoholism, beginning at age 16. Mrs. Jones reported that her father's drinking caused family problems and that he drank every night. There was no evidence of a psychiatric history in her brothers or her husband.

Mrs. Jones had a full-term male child who weighed 3,610 grams through a normal vaginal delivery. She was also on an antibiotic during the latter part of her pregnancy. Her son was hospitalized for 10 days following birth because of an elevated white blood count. She breastfed the baby and stayed in the hospital with him until day 8 postpartum. Mrs. Jones also noted that the baby experienced colic during at least the first 3 months postpartum.

About day 3 postpartum, Mrs. Jones' mood began to sink. She said that her low mood felt almost like physical pain. She also reported feeling anxious and irritable at this time. During the period of her depression, which lasted at least 2 months, she completely lost her appetite. She woke up during the night and could not get back to sleep. She commented that it was almost like not falling asleep. She had no energy and lost interest in most things. Mrs. Jones reported feeling guilty; in particular, she believed that she wasn't a good mother, and she blamed herself for her son's colic. She also had extreme difficulty in concentrating. Finally, she found that her work and family relationships were impaired by her depression. Despite both her mother and husband urging her to seek help for her depression, she did not. At 6 months postpartum, she was still reporting a moderate level of depressive symptomatology.

criteria used in many studies of postpartum depression, including our own study. What should also be apparent is that many of the somatic symptoms characterize normal women during the postpartum period. Problems such as fatigue and sleep difficulties may commonly be seen in the postpartum period. Researchers and clinicians need to be careful in interpreting the significance of these symptoms during the postpartum period. Many of the important characteristics of postpartum depression are found in Case History 1.3.

Prevalence

Blues

Studies of the prevalence of the blues have reported a wide range (O'Hara, 1991). Rates have ranged from 26% to 85% (Handley et al., 1980; O'Hara, 1987; O'Hara, Zekoski, Philipps, & Wright, 1990; Stein, Marsh, & Morton, 1981). Studies reporting relatively high prevalence rates have used rather liberal criteria, such as the presence of crying sometime during the first week after delivery (Harris, 1981; Stein et al., 1981; Yalom et al., 1968). Lower prevalence rates have been obtained in studies using more stringent criteria for the blues, such as high scores on standard depression or mood scales (Handley et al., 1980; O'Hara et al., 1990).

Several investigators have questioned whether blues symptoms are a specific response to childbirth or a more general response to any surgical procedure (Iles et al., 1989; Kendell, MacKenzie, West, McGuire, & Cox, 1984; Levy, 1987). Overall, studies that have addressed this question have found that childbearing women have blues symptoms that peak between 3 and 5 days after delivery, whereas female surgical patients show a general decline in symptom levels beginning shortly after surgery. Also, women undergoing major surgery tend to report higher symptom levels than childbearing women, particularly during the early postsurgical/postpartum period (Iles et al., 1989; Levy, 1987). The results of these studies suggest that a peaking of blues symptoms 3 to 5 days postpartum is a phenomenon specific to childbearing women.

Depression

Depression after childbirth would appear to be common (O'Hara & Zekoski, 1988). Early studies reported rates that ranged between 3% and 45% (Tod, 1964; Uddenberg, 1974). In general, the criteria used to define depression in these studies were unique to the study in question, making it difficult to compare prevalence rates across studies (O'Hara & Zekoski, 1988). It was not until the 1980s that investigators began to use diagnostic criteria (e.g., RDC) to define postpartum depression, and since that time the range of rates that have been reported in the United States and Europe has narrowed considerably.

Interestingly, both the lowest (7.3%) and highest (16.5%) rates of postpartum depression reported among adult women in North America have come from Canadian studies (Gotlib, Whiffen, Wallace, & Mount, 1991; Whiffen, 1988). Gotlib et al. (1991) followed up one of the largest samples to date (N = 730) and obtained a prevalence rate of 7.3% for major and minor depression at 5 weeks postpartum in London, Ontario. Whiffen's (1988) higher rate of depression (16.5%) was obtained from a sample recruited from a facility near Vancouver, British Columbia. In studies of primiparous women, Cutrona (1983) and Campbell and Cohn (1991) obtained similar rates of postpartum depression, 8.3% (based on DSM-III) and 9.3% (based on the RDC), respectively. In our first study at Iowa, we obtained a prevalence rate of 12% based on the RDC (O'Hara, Neunaber, & Zekoski, 1984). The only other study, with the exception of the one described in this volume, to obtain prevalence data based on diagnostic criteria was completed by Troutman and Cutrona (1990). They studied a sample of 128 pregnant adolescents (age range 14 to 18 years) and found a 26% prevalence rate of major and minor depression in the first 6 weeks postpartum (only 6% met criteria for major depression).

Similar rates of depression have been obtained in Great Britain when the diagnostic methods that were used were similar to those of North American studies. For example, Kumar and Robson (1984) obtained a prevalence of 14.9% for major and minor depression at 12 weeks postpartum, similar to the 12% rate reported by Watson et al. (1984) and the 10% rate reported by Wolkind, Coleman, and Ghodsian (1980) at 16 weeks postpartum. These studies were all conducted in London. Elsewhere in Great Britain, Cox, Connor, and Kendell (1982) reported a prevalence of 13% in the first 16 weeks postpartum, in a study conducted in Edinburgh. Nott (1987) obtained a prevalence rate of 18.5% at 12 weeks postpartum, based on a sample from Southampton; and Cooper, Campbell, Day, Kennerley, and Bond (1988) reported a prevalence of 8.7% in a sample from Cambridge. Based on the RDC, Carothers and Murray (1990) reported a prevalence of 12.6%, also using a Cambridge sample. Finally, a recent study conducted in Stoke-on-Trent (in the Midlands) found a 13.8% six-month period prevalence rate for postpartum depression based on the RDC (Cox, Murray, & Chapman, 1993). The range of depression rates observed in the British studies is remarkably similar to the range observed for the North American studies, particularly given that British investigators often classify women as psychiatric "cases" based on their level of impairment and secondarily identify a specific syndrome. As a result, it is likely that some of their cases would not meet RDC or DSM-III criteria for depression because of, for example, a predominance of anxiety symptoms.

Important questions have been raised recently regarding the extent to which depression is more prevalent during the postpartum period than at other times (i.e., during pregnancy or periods of nonchildbearing) (O'Hara, 1991). The study to be described in chapters 3 through 9 was largely designed to address these questions. Several studies have already addressed the relative risk of depression during the puerperium vs. pregnancy, and these studies have found that depression is more common after delivery, but not necessarily significantly so (O'Hara, 1991). For example, Kumar and Robson (1984) found an increased risk, ranging from 1.3 (relative to first trimester) to 5.3 (relative to second and third trimesters). Similar findings were obtained in other studies as well (e.g., Cox et al., 1982; Cutrona, 1983; O'Hara et al., 1984; Watson, et al. 1984). However, Gotlib, Whiffen, Mount, Milne, and Cordy, (1989) found a greater risk for depression during the second trimester than at 5 weeks postpartum. The major problem with most of these studies is that the period of time considered (for diagnosis) during pregnancy is often different from the period of time considered after delivery (e.g., Cox et al., 1982; O'Hara et al., 1984). The approach taken by Kumar and Robson (1984), in which they report rates of depression for consecutive 3-month periods (trimesters) beginning the trimester before pregnancy and continuing through the trimester after delivery, provides the clearest basis for comparing rates of depression during pregnancy with rates of depression after delivery. However, even the Kumar and Robson study did not statistically compare rates of depression across pregnancy and the puerperium, and so the question of whether depression is significantly more prevalent after delivery than during pregnancy remains unanswered.

Is the postpartum period a high-risk time for depression? This question had been addressed only indirectly prior to our study. Kumar and Robson (1984) reported that only 1 of their subjects had a new episode of depression in the 12 weeks before pregnancy, (the nonchildbearing control period) relative to 16 new episodes that occurred in the first 12 weeks after delivery (the postpartum period). However, Watson et al. (1984) noted that two recent studies of nonpuerperal women in nearby communities found, in one case, an equal prevalence of depression, and in the other case, a lower prevalence of depression compared to what they obtained in their own study of postpartum depression. Moreover, three more recent studies (two of which were initiated about the time of the current study) found little evidence of increased risk of depression during the puerperium. Cooper et al. (1988) compared rates of depression in a sample of childbearing subjects from Cambridge and a sample of sociodemographically similar subjects from Edinburgh and found no differences. In another British study, Cox et al. (1993) found equivalent rates of depression (over the first 6 months postpartum) in large samples of childbearing and matched nonchildbearing control subjects; however, the childbearing women did show a significantly higher rate of depression relative to the matched controls in the first five weeks postpartum. Troutman and Cutrona (1990) compared relatively matched samples of adolescent childbearing and nonchildbearing subjects in a prospective design and found no significant differences in rates of depression. Again, the Kumar and Robson study (1984) provides the best evidence that risk for depression may increase during the puerperium. However, other studies, more contemporaneous with our own, cast doubt on that premise.

One index of severity of depression is the length of the episode. In general, it would appear that postpartum depressions persist over several months (O'Hara, 1991). Depicted in Figure 1.1 is a graphical description of onset and duration depressions during pregnancy and the puerperium from Watson et al. (1984). They reported that one-quarter of their depressed subjects had episodes lasting 3 months or more and another quarter had episodes lasting 6 months or more. Also, Kumar, and Robson (1984) found that 50% of their depressed subjects had episodes lasting 6 months or more. Several other British studies obtained essentially the same results (Cox, Rooney, Thomas, & Wrate, 1984; Pitt, 1968; Wolkind et al., 1980). Campbell, Cohn, Flanagan, Popper, and Myers (1992) reported an average duration of 15 weeks, with many other women experiencing ongoing symptoms at a subclinical level. Only our earlier study (O'Hara et al., 1984) reported a rather short average length of postpartum episodes, 3.1 weeks; however, we followed up only until 9 weeks postpartum.

Causal Factors

Postpartum depression has increasingly come to be defined in terms of diagnostic criteria such as the RDC (Spitzer et al., 1978). The prevalence estimates for depression described earlier in this chapter were largely based on RDC-defined depression. However, studies that have investigated correlates or causal factors in postpartum depression have often used indices that measure severity of depression (O'Hara, 1991). Examples of these measures would include the Beck Depression Inventory (Beck, Ward, Mendelson, Mock, & Erbaugh, 1961), the Depression Adjective Checklist (Lubin, 1965), the Multiple Affective Adjective Checklist (Zuckerman & Lubin, 1965), the Edinburgh Postnatal Depression Scale (Cox, Holden, & Sagovsky, 1987), and a variety of visual analogue scales (Kendell et al., 1984). These measures, which are used to index mood at the time of completion, may be administered at any time during the puerperium and may be taken to reflect severity of postpartum depression or the blues. However, the relationship between a score on a mood measure and a diagnosis of postpartum depression is usually unclear, making it difficult to generalize from studies defining depression on the basis of a severity measure to the phenomenon of postpartum depression (defined diagnostically). Moreover, in these studies, particularly those in which hormonal variables are examined, little distinction is made between symptoms of depression and symptoms of the blues. For this reason studies of causal factors in the blues and depression have been combined in one section.

Background Factors

There is little evidence that demographic characteristics are associated with increased risk for the blues or depression (O'Hara, 1991). Having few financial resources and caring for a first child are examples of factors that might be expected to increase the stressfulness of the puerperium and to increase a woman's risk for blues or depression (Brown & Harris, 1978), but there is little evidence that these factors are associated with increased risk for postpartum blues or depression. The relationships between risk for postpartum blues/depression and background factors such as age, socioeconomic status (SES), education level, parity, and marital status have been observed in a number of studies (O'Hara, 1991; O'Hara & Zekoski, 1988). In the many studies that have been conducted, there is almost no evidence that any particular background characteristic puts a woman at increased risk for postpartum depression. For example, in 18 studies that have examined the relationship between parity and postpartum depression, no relationship was found in 12 studies, higher levels of parity were associated with increased risk for postpartum depression in 3 studies, and lower levels of parity were associated with increased risk for postpartum depression in 3 studies (O'Hara & Zekoski, 1988). What remains to be done with respect to the possible role of demographic factors, particularly given the evidence linking low SES to depression in young women, is a quantitative analysis (i.e., a meta-analysis) that would provide estimates of the effect sizes of the correlations between the various sociodemographic variables and postpartum depression and the blues (Spangler, 1992).

Biological Factors

Many hypotheses accounting for the biological basis of postpartum blues and depression have been tested in a large number of studies, particularly over the past 15 years. Interest in a biological etiology is in part due to the dramatic hormonal changes that occur in women during the first few days after delivery. Levels of progesterone, estradiol, and free estriol drop dramatically, on the order of 90% to 95% (Speroff, Glass, & Kase, 1989). Also, these changes occur during a period when many women report symptoms of the postpartum blues. For these reasons hormonal factors have been thought to play an important etiologic role in postpartum mood disorders (O'Hara, 1991). For example, it has been hypothesized that levels of hormones such as the estrogens, progesterone, prolactin, and cortisol are too high or too low in the puerperium or that changes in the levels of these hormones occur too quickly or not quickly enough (Stein, 1982). The hormonal dysfunction hypothesis is similar to that proposed for mood disturbances in the premenstrual period and during menopause (Yalom et al., 1968; Carroll & Steiner, 1978; Dalton, 1980). In addition, numerous biological hypotheses derived from the more general depression literature have been tested in childbearing women. Studies testing biological hypotheses will be reviewed selectively, emphasizing hormonal variables that we included in our own study (i.e., progesterone, estrogens, cortisol, and prolactin). Comprehensive reviews of this literature can be found in George and Sandler (1988) and Hamilton and Harberger (1992).

Steroid Hormones

Progesterone

Progesterone withdrawal has been hypothesized as a causal factor in postpartum mood disorders (Dalton, 1980). The evidence for this hypothesis has been decidedly mixed (O'Hara, 1991), with only two studies providing any support (Harris et al., 1989; Nott, Franklin, Armitage, & Gelder, 1976). In a sample of 27 women, Nott et al. (1976) found a significant association between magnitude of decline in progesterone after delivery (between roughly week 38 gestation and day 1 postpartum) and depressed mood in the first week postpartum. In a later and more sophisticated study, which was based on assessments conducted at about 8 weeks postpartum, Harris et al. (1989) reported lower levels of progesterone among depressed breast-feeding women than among nondepressed breast-feeding women. Among the bottle-feeding women, just the opposite association was observed. Several other studies of the postpartum blues failed to find any association between progesterone levels and mood (Ballinger, Kay, Naylor, & Smith, 1982; Kuevi et al., 1983; Metz et al., 1983). One study did find significantly higher levels of progesterone in 5 women experiencing the blues as compared to 5 symptom-free women (Feksi, Harris, Walker, Riad-Fahmy, & Newcombe, 1984).

Estrogens

Estrogen levels, much like progesterone levels, decrease markedly after childbirth. Several studies have investigated the relationship between estrogen levels (usually estradiol) and postpartum blues and depression. Most of these studies have produced negative findings (Gard, Handley, Parsons, & Waldron, 1986; Harris et al., 1989; Kuevi et al., 1983; Metz et al., 1983). Nott et al. (1976) found lower levels of total estrogen prior to delivery among women who experienced the blues in the first week postpartum, and Feksi et al. (1984) found higher levels of estradiol among women who experienced the blues in the first week postpartum. Despite these negative findings, there has been a recent interest in estrogen-based prophylaxis of postpartum depression (Henderson, Gregoire, Kumar, & Studd, 1991).

Cortisol

Abnormalities in the hypothalamic–pituitary–adrenal system have been studied intensively as etiologic factors in major depression (Schlesser, 1986). Both free and bound cortisol are elevated during late pregnancy, peak at high levels during labor, drop precipitously after delivery to about late pregnancy levels, and gradually decline over a period of time (Jolivet, Blanchier, & Gautray, 1974). Both overproduction and sudden withdrawal of corticosteroids have been posited as potential causes of postpartum mood disorders (George & Sandler, 1988; Railton, 1961). Studies testing these hypotheses have yielded very few positive results with respect to either postpartum blues or depression (Feksi et al., 1984; Harris et al., 1989; Kuevi et al., 1983). Handley et al. (1980) did find significantly higher levels of cortisol at 38 weeks gestation in women who later experienced the postpartum blues than in women who did not; however, they did not replicate this finding in a later study (Gard et al., 1986). Ballinger et al. (1982) reported significantly higher urinary levels of 11-hydroxycortisol steroids on day 1 after delivery in a group of women who showed the greatest amount of increased positive mood between days 2 and 4 postpartum. Ehlert, Patalla, Kirschbaum, Piedmont, and Hellhammer (1990) found significantly higher morning levels of salivary cortisol in women with the postpartum blues on days when their symptoms were "severe" than in women without the blues. Finally, disturbances in cortisol dynamics, reflected in dexamethasone nonsuppression, do not appear to distinguish postpartum-depressed and -nondepressed women in the early puerperium (Greenwood & Parker, 1984; Singh et al., 1986).

Peptide Hormones

Prolactin

The final hormone that we investigated in our study was prolactin. Levels of prolactin, which are very high by the end of pregnancy, fall more slowly after delivery than the gonadal hormones. In nonchildbearing women very high levels of prolactin (hyperprolactinemia) are associated with depression, anxiety, and hostility (Campbell & Winokur, 1985). As with the steroid hormones, the findings for prolactin have been mixed. Daily basal levels of plasma prolactin have been found to be positively correlated with daily measures of dysphoric mood on days 2, 4, and 6 postpartum (George, Copeland, & Wilson, 1980). In contrast, a more recent study reported that lower levels of prolactin were associated with higher levels of depression at 8 weeks postpartum (Harris et al., 1989).

Other studies have found no association between postpartum mood and prolactin levels (e.g., Nott et al., 1976). It should be noted that prolactin is a difficult hormone to measure well in the puerperium. Breast feeding stimulates prolactin secretion, and prolactin levels are significantly higher in breast-feeding women than in non-breast-feeding women (Vemer & Rolland, 1981). There has also been a suggestion in the literature that even slight ambulation stimulates prolactin secretion (George & Sandler, 1988); however, we have found little evidence of this phenomenon (O'Hara, Schlechte, Lewis, & Uacner, 1991).

Other Biological Variables

In addition to progesterone, the estrogens, cortisol, and prolactin, which were hormones that we studied in our investigation, other biological variables, including β-endorphin (Brimsmead, Smith, Singh, Lewin, & Owens, 1982), electrolytes (Stein et al., 1981), vitamins (Livingston et al., 1978), and thyroid dysfunction (George & Wilson, 1983; Harris et al., 1989; Pop et al., 1991) have been studied as potential contributors to postpartum blues and depression. Of these biological variables, tryptophan and thyroid dysfunction deserve special comment.

Plasma Tryptophan

Tryptophan is a precursor of serotonin (5-HT) and has been studied in postpartum mood disorders on the assumption that an inadequate supply of the 5-HT precursor tryptophan might result in inadequate release of 5-HT. Moreover, recent research has implicated serotonin dysregulation in the etiology of major depression (Mann et al., 1992). Several early studies obtained results in support of a potential role for lowered levels of tryptophan in postpartum mood disorders. Stein, Milton, Bebbington, Wood, and Coppen (1976) reported a significant negative correlation between free tryptophan levels and postpartum depression at 6 days postpartum. A similar finding was reported by Handley, Dunn, Baker, Cockshoff, and Gould (1977). In a much larger study, Handley et al. (1980) found that total tryptophan recovered to its normal higher level more quickly after delivery in women not experiencing the blues than in women experiencing the blues. There were no differences for free tryptophan. Finally, Harris (1980) conducted a double-blind, placebo-controlled study of the effects of 3 g of L-tryptophan per day for 10 days on the development of the postpartum blues in a sample of 55 women. Supplementary tryptophan did not reduce the incidence of the blues.

Thyroid Dysfunction

Hamilton (1962) has argued that hypothyroidism may be a cause of postpartum depression, particularly when it begins more than 2 weeks after delivery. However, neither Grimmell and Larsen (1965) nor George and Wilson (1983) found evidence of any association between thyroid function or thyroid levels and postpartum mood disturbance. More positive findings were obtained in two recent studies. Harris et al. (1989) reported an association between depression-meeting DSM-III criteria and thyroid dysfunction (either hyper- or hypothyroidism) measured at 6 weeks postpartum. Similarly, Pop et al. (1991) found a significant association between depression meeting the RDC criteria and thyroid dysfunction (either hyper- or hypothyroidism) at one of several assessments during the first 34 weeks postpartum.

There has been little consistency in the findings of studies of hormonal variables. One major problem with this research has been the inconsistency with which postpartum mood has been measured and the timing of those measurements. This problem is common to all of the research on postpartum depression. A second major problem is that the simple hormonal models are unable to account for much variability in postpartum mood. There may be many reasons for this state of affairs. For example, the wrong hormones may have been studied; or the complex interrelationships among hormones, neurotransmitters, and other biological factors may not have been adequately captured. Finally, hormonal factors may only be important for women who are otherwise vulnerable to affective disorder. This vulnerability could be in itself biological/genetic (e.g., reflected in a personal or family history of affective disorders) in nature. It could also be psychological (e.g., poor cognitive/social coping with stress) or social/environmental (e.g., poor marital relationship, adverse social circumstances). Obviously, all three of these possibilities may be true; the potential roles of these other factors are reviewed in the next several sections.

Gynecologic and Obstetric Factors

Links between menstrual problems and postpartum mood disturbance have been hypothesized by several investigators (e.g., Yalom et al., 1968; Steiner, 1979) based on the assumption that similar types of hormonal dysfunction might underlie both premenstrual and postpartum mood disorders. For example, one study (Dennerstein, Morse, & Varnavides, 1988) compared women with prospectively determined premenstrual syndrome and women with no menstrual problems and found only a marginally higher rate of past postpartum depression among the women with premenstrual syndrome. Several other studies have reported significant associations between "premenstrual tension" and the postpartum blues (Nott et al., 1976; Playfair & Gowers, 1981; Yalom et al., 1968). However, none of these reports provided any description of their criteria for "premenstrual tension." Also, painful menstruation (dysmenorrhea) has been found to be associated with postpartum mood disturbance

(Jacobson, Kaij, & Nilsson, 1965; Pitt, 1968; Playfair & Gowers, 1981). However, Uddenberg (1974) found that women who experienced either much or no pain during menstruation reported high levels of postpartum symptoms, and Nilsson and Almgren (1970) found no relationship between postpartum symptoms and severity of dysmenorrhea.

Obstetric complications, which could be considered as stressful life events, have been inconsistently related to postpartum depression, with some studies finding less mood disturbance in women with more stress or delivery complications (O'Hara et al., 1982; Paykel, Emms, Fletcher, & Rassaby, 1980; Pitt, 1968). Other studies have found the expected relationship between obstetric complications and postpartum mood disturbance (Campbell & Cohn, 1991; Hannah, Adams, Lee, Glover, & Sandler, 1992; Oakley, 1980; O'Hara et al., 1984; Tod, 1964), and still others have found no association (Cox et al., 1982; Playfair & Gowers, 1981; Dalton, 1971). Finally, previous abortion or miscarriage has been inconsistently associated with postpartum mood. Although two studies did find an association (Playfair & Gowers, 1981; Jacobson et al., 1965), several did not (Paykel et al., 1980; Kumar & Robson, 1984; Watson et al., 1984).

The variability in the outcomes of studies of the effects of obstetric stress is in part due to the various measures of stress that have been used. For example, O'Hara et al. (1982) found that women who experienced more stressful deliveries (with caesarean section defined as most stressful) reported lower levels of postpartum depressive symptomatology. One possible explanation for this counterintuitive finding is that certain obstetric events (e.g., caesarean section) are cues for the social environment to provide high levels of postpartum support or help that more than compensate for the stressful event. Findings such as this emphasize the importance of considering variables, such as social support, that may ameliorate the effects of obstetric and nonobstetric stress in the puerperium.

Stressful Life Events

Negative life events (e.g., serious illness in a family member; unemployment), which have been found to increase the likelihood of depression in nonpuerperal women (Brown & Harris, 1978; Paykel, 1979), may occur during pregnancy and after delivery. Negative events might be especially potent during this period if they have implications for the woman's ability to care properly for her infant (e.g., severe financial reversal, abandonment by spouse). Not surprisingly, a number of studies have found that higher levels of stressful life events during pregnancy and after delivery were associated with higher levels of postpartum depression symptoms (O'Hara et al., 1982; Cutrona, 1983; O'Hara et al., 1984; Playfair &

Gowers, 1981), an increased probability of a clinical postpartum depression (Martin, Brown, Goldberg, & Brockington, 1989; O'Hara, 1986; O'Hara, Rehm, & Campbell, 1983; Paykel et al., 1980), and higher risk for relapse after delivery among women with previous histories of affective disorder (Marks, Wieck, Checkley, & Kumar, 1992). There have been some failures to find the expected association between negative life events and depression (Hopkins, Campbell, & Marcus, 1987; Kumar & Robson, 1984; Pitt, 1968), however, in one of the studies, the investigators did find an association between infant postnatal complications and postpartum depression (Hopkins et al., 1987). Nevertheless, all of these studies taken as a whole suggest an important role for negative life events in postpartum depression.

Marital Relationship

Probably no relationship is more important to a woman during the puerperium than that with her husband. Many studies have found that postpartum-depressed women report poor marital relationships after delivery (Campbell et al., 1992; Cox et al., 1982; Martin, 1977; O'Hara et al., 1983; Paykel et al., 1980); although one recent study found no differences between depressed and nondepressed women (Hopkins et al., 1987). More importantly, several studies assessed the marital relationship during pregnancy and found that the poor marital relationship preceded the postpartum depression (Braverman & Roux, 1978; Gotlib et al., 1991; Kumar & Robson, 1984; O'Hara, 1986; Robinson, Olmsted, & Garner, 1989; Watson et al., 1984; Whiffen, 1988). However, in a few studies, it has been found that marital distress during pregnancy did not predict postpartum depression (O'Hara et al., 1983; Blair, Gilmore, Playfair, Tisdall, & O'Shea, 1970) or depression relapse during the puerperium (Marks et al., 1992).

Parental Conflict

A few investigators have studied the effect of parental conflict and loss on the likelihood of postpartum depression. Several studies found that a poor mother–daughter relationship was associated with postpartum depression (Kumar & Robson, 1984; Nilsson & Almgren, 1970; Uddenberg, 1974). In a recent study, Gotlib et al. (1991) found that more negative perceptions measured during pregnancy of maternal and paternal caring during childhood were associated with diagnosis of postpartum depression. However, Paykel et al. (1980) found no association between parental conflict or childhood parental loss and postpartum depression. Similarly, Watson et al. (1984) found no association between childhood separation from parents and postpartum depression.

Social Support

Social support from spouse, family, and friends during times of stress (e.g., helping in household tasks, acting as a confidant) is thought to reduce the likelihood of depression (Mueller, 1980). The findings from research linking social support and postpartum depression have been rather consistent. Lack of support from the spouse has been found to be associated with increased levels of postpartum depression (Blair et al., 1970; Campbell et al., 1992; Feggetter & Gath, 1981; O'Hara, 1986; O'Hara et al., 1983); however, Hopkins et al. (1987) failed to replicate this finding. Other studies have found that lack of an adequate confidant or lower levels of support from a confidant are associated with postpartum depression (O'Hara et al., 1983; Paykel et al., 1980). Finally, Cutrona (1984) reported that several dimensions of perceived social support measured during pregnancy were associated with level of postpartum depression symptoms.

Personal and Family Psychopathology

Indices of depressive symptomatology, anxiety, and neurotic behavior during pregnancy have been consistently associated with level of postpartum depressive symptomatology and have been found to distinguish postpartum-depressed and -nondepressed women (Cutrona, 1983; Dalton, 1971; Hayworth et al., 1980; Nilsson & Almgren, 1970; O'Hara et al., 1984; O'Hara et al., 1982; Playfair & Gowers, 1981; Watson et al., 1984). Although the general pattern of these findings have been very consistent and may indicate a continuity of psychological distress across pregnancy and the puerperium, a few studies have found little association between pre- and postpartum distress (Kumar & Robson, 1984).

Women who have experienced previous psychiatric disorder would appear to be at risk for postpartum depression. Several studies have obtained data regarding previous psychiatric disturbance and found an association with postpartum depression (Campbell et al., 1992; Jacobson et al., 1965; Martin, 1977; Nilsson & Almgren, 1970; O'Hara et al., 1983; Paykel et al., 1980; Playfair & Gowers, 1981; Tod, 1964; Uddenberg, 1974; Watson et al., 1984). A recent study that included women with previous histories of bipolar disorder, schizoaffective disorder, or major depression found that 22 of the 43 women (51%) experienced a psychotic or nonpsychotic depression or mania (and, in a few cases, an anxiety disorder) after delivery. However, at least four studies have not found the expected association between psychiatric history and postpartum depression (Blair et al., 1970; Dalton, 1971; Kumar & Robson, 1984; Pitt, 1968). Also in an earlier study (O'Hara, 1986), we had reported that number of previous episodes of depression was associated with risk for postpartum depression; however, that effect was largely due to one subject who had numerous episodes and cannot be considered reliable.

Family history of psychopathology has also been studied as a predictor of postpartum depression in a few studies. The findings from these studies have largely been supportive of an association between family psychopathology and postpartum depression (Campbell et al., 1992; Nilsson & Almgren, 1970; O'Hara et al., 1984; Watson et al., 1984), although not uniformly so (Kumar & Robson, 1984). This issue was one of the major questions that we addressed in our own study.

Psychological Constructs

Several constructs derived from cognitive–behavioral theories of depression (Abramson, Seligman, & Teasdale, 1978; Beck, Rush, Shaw, & Emery, 1979; Lewinsohn, Youngren, & Grosscup, 1979; Rehm, 1977) have been tested as predictors of postpartum depression. The logic of these studies was that certain types of psychological vulnerability, such as dysfunctional attributional style or self-control attitudes, or maladaptive cognitions, should increase a person's risk for depression in the context of a stressful life event (e.g., giving birth). For example, O'Hara et al. (1982) and Cutrona (1983) found that attributional style (the types of causes women identify for good and bad events) (Abramson et al., 1978) measured during pregnancy predicted level of postpartum depression; however, other studies failed to replicate these results (Manly et al., 1982; O'Hara et al., 1984; Whiffen, 1988). O'Hara et al. (1982) found that subjects' attitudes about self-control (Rehm, 1977), measured during pregnancy, were significantly correlated with postpartum depression level but were not significant in a regression equation predicting postpartum depression level.

In a later study (O'Hara et al., 1984), self-control attitudes were found to be significant in a regression equation predicting postpartum depression level but not postpartum depression diagnosis. Finally, a few studies have tested Beck's cognitive model of depression (Beck et al., 1979) with mixed results (Gotlib et al., 1991; O'Hara et al., 1982) and Lewinsohn's behavioral model (Atkinson & Rickel, 1984; O'Hara et al., 1982) with generally supportive results.

Summary

None of the potential social and psychological causal factors in postpartum depression have been supported unambiguously in the literature. The pattern of results reviewed here would suggest that gynecologic and obstetric variables are not specifically related to postpartum depression. There is good evidence that a woman's psychological adjustment before and during pregnancy and, to a lesser extent, a history of family psychopathology are associated with the development of postpartum depression.

Moreover, women who experience high levels of stress during pregnancy and after delivery as well as women who lack a supportive spouse would appear to be particularly vulnerable to developing postpartum depression. These are psychosocial variables that figure very prominently in models of nonpostpartum depression (Depue, 1979). In fact, many recent investigators have assumed that the postpartum period is simply a high-risk time for depression and that it is an appropriate context in which to test etiologic models developed to account for nonpostpartum depression (Atkinson & Rickel, 1984; Cutrona, 1983; Gotlib et al., 1991; O'Hara et al., 1982; Whiffen, 1988).

Consequences

Postpartum mood disorders may have negative consequences for the woman herself, her child(ren), and the family. Most of the research that has been done in this area has addressed the issue of depression relapse/recurrence in the postpartum-depressed mother and the short- and long-term consequences of maternal depression for the child. Very little research has addressed the issue of possible negative consequences of the blues. Its most serious consequence may be that it heralds a later, more serious postpartum depression (Paykel et al., 1980). Even this consequence was not replicated in a more recent study (Gard et al., 1986). There have been no studies of the consequences of the blues to the child or family; however, the transient nature of the blues would suggest that even short-term negative consequences would be few.

For the Mother

Five long-term follow-up studies of women participating in postpartum depression projects have been reported (Cox et al., 1984; Ghodsian, Zajicek, & Wolkind, 1984; Kumar & Robson, 1984; Philipps & O'Hara, 1991; Uddenberg & Englesson, 1978). Overall, these studies have found that postpartum-depressed women followed up over periods ranging from 1 to $4\frac{1}{2}$ years after delivery were more likely to be depressed than women who earlier had not experienced a postpartum depression. For example, Kumar and Robson (1984) followed up 99 of 119 women 4 years after delivery. They found that 6 of 14 women who had experienced a new episode of depression at 3 months postpartum continued to seek psychiatric assistance in the intervening 4 years. Our own study (Philipps & O'Hara, 1991), described in detail in chapter 2, yielded similar findings. These follow-up studies suggest that at any length of follow-up, women who have experienced a postpartum depression are at increased risk for depression.

For the Child

A large number of studies have investigated the consequences to the child of having a mother who experienced a postpartum depression. The short-term studies generally have evaluated the child at a few months of age while the woman was still depressed (Cohn, Campbell, Matias, & Hopkins, 1990; Field et al., 1988; Field, Sandberg, Garcia, Vega-Lahr, Goldstein, & Guy, 1985; Whiffen & Gotlib, 1989). Longer-term follow-up studies have evaluated children up to age $4\frac{1}{2}$; mothers were not necessarily depressed at the time (Cogill, Caplan, Alexandra, Robson, & Kumar, 1986; Ghodsian et al., 1984; Kumar & Robson, 1984; Murray, 1992; Philipps & O'Hara, 1991; Stein et al., 1991; Uddenberg & Englesson, 1978). The results of these studies have not been uniform, but in general they suggest that depressed mothers are more negative in their interactions with their infants and that older children (up to age $4\frac{1}{2}$) show social and cognitive deficits relative to children of women who had not experienced a postpartum depression.

Representative of the short-term follow-up studies is one conducted by Cohn et al. (1990). They observed 24 depressed and 22 nondepressed mother–infant dyads at 2 months postpartum, in both structured and unstructured interactions. They found that depressed mothers showed higher levels of negative affect, primarily irritation and intrusiveness, during the face-to-face interactions. Also, the babies of the depressed nonworking mothers showed a lower proportion of positive affect than the babies of nondepressed mothers and depressed mothers who worked.

A long-term follow-up study was conducted by Kumar and his colleagues. At the age of 4 years, 94 children of women who had participated in a study of postpartum depression (Kumar & Robson, 1984) were evaluated on measures of cognitive abilities and social and emotional development. Children of women who had experienced a postpartum depression performed significantly worse on the McCarthy scales of children's (cognitive) abilities than children of women who did not experience a postpartum depression (Cogill et al., 1986); however, there were no differences between the two groups of children with respect to their social and emotional development (Caplan et al., 1989). Other studies have found a significant association between postpartum depression and later social and emotional problems in the children (Wrate, Rooney, Thomas, & Cox, 1985), reflecting the mix of findings in this area as well as in others.

Treatment Studies

A wide variety of psychological and pharmacological treatments for postpartum depression have been evaluated. Unfortunately, very few of these studies meet contemporary standards for treatment research. Many of the treatments have been aimed at preventing postpartum mood disorders, while others target women who are already depressed (Gordon & Gordon, 1960; Holden, Sagovsky, & Cox, 1989).

Prevention

In a seminal study, Gordon and Gordon (1960) evaluated a 2-session prenatal group intervention aimed at providing women (or couples) with practical advice to reduce postpartum emotional distress. Examples of advice given in the group sessions included "The responsibilities of being a mother (and not a martyr) are learned, hence get help and advice." "Don't give up your outside interests, but cut down the responsibilities and rearrange your schedules" (p. 434). The authors found that women who attended these groups, particularly those who attended with their spouses, experienced significantly less emotional distress after delivery than women who did not attend these group sessions.

Halonen and Passman (1985) reported on a study of prenatal preparation in which they assigned 48 pregnant women who had received labor-specific relaxation training to 1 of 4 groups: (1) additional relaxation training; (2) extended relaxation training that emphasized possible postpartum stressors; (3) discussion of postpartum stressors; and (4) a control discussion about their awareness of postpartum stress. They found that the groups receiving relaxation training were significantly less distressed than the nonrelaxation training groups during the first 9 weeks postpartum. They also found that the groups that discussed possible postpartum stressors were less elated after delivery than the groups not exposed. The authors recommended the use of extended nonspecific relaxation training both before and after delivery as a way of reducing postpartum emotional distress.

Elliott, Sanjack, and Leverton (1988) evaluated the efficacy of prenatal groups for women who were at risk for postpartum depression on the basis of having been treated for a prior depression, having a poor marital relationship, lacking a confidant, or having a high level of anxiety during pregnancy. These women, who were considered to be at high risk, were expected to have about a 3-fold increased risk for a postpartum depression. The group sessions were psychoeducational; and to a large degree, the participants were free to influence the course of the meetings, 5 of which occurred during pregnancy and 6 of which occurred after delivery on a monthly basis. The findings were that women who participated in these groups were significantly less likely than the women who did not receive the treatment to experience a depression at 3 months postpartum.

In a recent study, Wolman, Chalmers, Hofmeyr, and Nikodem (1993) evaluated the efficacy of providing companionship during labor to a group of women who had no companions of their own. The authors reasoned that labor was a time when women were especially vulnerable to losing confidence in their competence as mothers and that feelings of incompetence as a mother was a causal factor in the development of postpartum depression. The provision of support during labor was hypothesized to increase women's confidence in their competence and to reduce depressive and anxious symptomatology during the postpartum period. This rather brief intervention during labor resulted in significantly greater levels of confidence and significantly lower levels of postpartum depressive and anxious symptomatology in the treated group relative to the untreated group.

Finally, in an uncontrolled trial of progesterone, 100 women who had at least 1 previous episode of postpartum depression were treated with 7 days of 100 mg intramuscularly administered progesterone and followed that with 60 days of 400 mg progesterone suppositories twice a day (Dalton, 1985). She reported a 10% recurrence rate of postpartum depression within six months of delivery which compares favorably with Dalton's expected recurrence rate of 68%. However, the lack of a control group and other methodological problems make these findings difficult to interpret.

Treatment

Relatively few controlled treatment trials for postpartum depression have been undertaken. The most adequate to date was one undertaken by Holden et al. (1989). Health visitors in Scotland offered 8 one-half-hour client-centered counseling sessions to 26 women meeting RDC for major depression. Compared to the 24 women who did not receive the intervention, the treated women had significantly lower levels of depressive symptomatology at the time of the posttherapy assessment. In a Canadian study, postpartum-depressed women (based on self-report) received 8 group sessions of social support group therapy or no treatment (Fleming, Klein, & Corter, 1992). There were no treatment effects with respect to depressive symptomatology; however, there was some evidence that the social support groups had a positive effect on mother–infant interaction.

Very little work on the pharmacotherapy of postpartum depression has been carried out. One British study evaluated the effects of transdermal estrogen in a double-blind, randomized, placebo-controlled study (Henderson et al., 1991). Preliminary results suggested that women receiving 6 months of treatment with estradiol skin patches showed a more rapid improvement in their depressive symptomatology than women in the placebo condition. Nevertheless, there was some question regarding the overall effectiveness of the estrogen treatment.

Summary

Postpartum mood disorders are relatively common, in part because the childbearing years encompass the period during which women are most at risk for depression. Fortunately, the most severe of these disorders (psychosis) is relatively uncommon and the most common of these disorders (the blues) is not disabling. Nevertheless, depression is relatively common and has serious consequences for women and their families. A large variety of social, environmental, and biological causes have been posited for postpartum mood disorders, many of which seem to be associated with depression that occurs at other times and in other contexts. Relatively few specific treatments for postpartum mood disorders have been developed and evaluated. The work described in the rest of this volume represents the attempts by our group to begin to address several of the major unresolved questions regarding the prevalence, causes, and consequences of postpartum mood disorders.

2
Preliminary Work

The history of psychological research on postpartum depression in North America has been strongly tied to research on cognitive and behavioral models of depression (e.g., Beck, 1970; Lewinsohn et al., 1979). In the late 1970s, the behavioral, cognitive, learned helplessness, and self-control models of depression were all being subjected to numerous experimental tests using cross-sectional designs and college-student subjects (e.g., Craighead, Hickey, & DeMonbreun, 1979; Klein, Fencil-Morse, & Seligman, 1976). Most studies were attempting to link deficits proposed by the various depression models to the presence (or severity) of depression, usually indexed by self-report measures such as the Beck Depression Inventory. Two major limitations of this research led to an interest in studies of postpartum depression.

The major problem in cross-sectional studies was that it was especially difficult to establish causal precedence for the presumed etiological variables proposed by the various depression models. This limitation of correlational research was particularly acute given that some of the proposed causal factors were similar to symptoms of depression. For example, the cognitive model (Beck et al., 1979, pp. 11–12) proposes that a "negative view of the self," part of the negative cognitive triad, is causally related to depression even though it could just as easily be viewed simply as a symptom of depression. A second problem was the concern that findings from research conducted with college students would not generalize to other populations.

The prospective study of childbearing women seemed to offer a solution to some of the problems of earlier research on cognitive and behavioral models of depression. First, the postpartum period was thought to be a time during which women were at high risk for becoming depressed (Paykel et al., 1980). One of the difficulties of prospective studies of psychopathology has been the need to follow large samples of subjects in order to have enough cases for a reasonably powerful design. Estimates of the prevalence of postpartum depression in the late 1970s were quite variable but ranged from about 10% to above 20%. These prevalence rates suggested that a prospective study would be feasible. A second advantage of studying childbearing women was that the period of risk was reasonably well defined (or so it was thought). Childbirth as a stressful life event was predictable and clearly defined in time; and the postpartum period, although a more ambiguous concept, was often defined as lasting between 6 and 12 weeks after delivery. These characteristics of childbearing women made prospective studies of depression feasible.

Postpartum Depression I: Tests of Cognitive–Behavioral Models

The major purpose of the first study in our series (O'Hara *et al.*, 1982; 1983) was to test the adequacy of several cognitive–behavioral depression models in accounting for depressive symptomatology during the postpartum period. These models included (1) the cognitive model (Beck, 1970); (2) the learned helplessness/attributional model (Abramson et al., 1978); (3) the behavioral model (Lewinsohn et al., 1979); and (4) the self-control model (Rehm, 1977). The presumed depression vulnerability factors proposed by each of the models, which are described below, were assessed with self-report measures during pregnancy.

The cognitive model (Beck, 1972) posits that beliefs reflecting a negative view of the self, world, and future lead directly to symptoms of depression such as low self-esteem, disturbed interpersonal relationships, and pessimism. These beliefs, often called the *negative cognitive triad,* are presumed to be caused by faulty information processing due to idiosyncratic schemas that developed early in life. For example, a person who experienced a painful loss as a child might have a schema regarding loss that is very broad, so any sort of a loss, no matter how trivial, is encoded as a significant negative event. This encoding, in turn, may activate the negative cognitive triad and lead to depression.

The learned helplessness/attributional model (Abramson et al., 1978) posits that internal (e.g., "This failure is my fault"), stable (e.g., "I always fail when I do this"), and global (e.g., "I fail at everything I try") attributions for past or present noncontingency (often negative events such as a failure or loss) would lead to the expectation of future noncontingency and consequently to symptoms of helplessness/depression. Attributional style—the predisposition of a person to make certain types of attributions for events—is believed to play an important role in vulnerability to depression. In this study we examined the attributional style of subjects as a predictor of postpartum depression.

The behavioral model (Lewinsohn et al., 1979) posits that a reduced level of response-contingent positive reinforcement leads to the symptoms of depression. Examples of this type of reduction or loss would include the retired couple who move to a new community away from family and friends and experience the loss of their normal sources of social reinforcement. A woman staying home to care for a new baby, thereby reducing contact with friends and colleagues from work, might have a similar experience.

The self-control model (Rehm, 1977) posits that a disturbance in self-regulation leads to symptoms of depression. Self-control is characterized by three interrelated processes: self-monitoring, self-evaluation, and self-reinforcement. Examples of disturbances to these processes include paying excessive attention to one's failures and shortcomings (negative self-monitoring) and setting standards that are excessively stringent (negative self-evaluation).

We were also interested in the extent to which stressful life events in addition to childbirth increased the risk of depressive symptomatology. By the end of the 1970s, there was a rather large literature linking stressful life events with depression (Brown & Harris, 1978). It was easy to imagine that stressful events occurring during pregnancy or during the early postpartum period would be more difficult than usual to handle well because of the physical effects of pregnancy and the later demands of caring for a new baby.

Social support from family members and confidants was believed to provide a buffer against the negative effects of stressful life events for the new mother and to reduce the likelihood of postpartum depression (Mueller, 1980; O'Hara et al., 1983). Earlier work had suggested that support provided by a spouse and a confidant were especially important (Brown & Harris, 1978), so we assessed support provided by these individuals and the women's parents as well.

Subjects

A total of 170 of 226 women initially recruited for the study completed it. Subjects were recruited during the second trimester of pregnancy from a public obstetrics and gynecology clinic and two private practices. The mean age of subjects was 26.6 years; the mean education level was 13.9 grades. Eighty-seven percent of subjects were white, 85.3% were married, and 45% were childless. Of the 56 subjects who failed to complete the study, 30 did not complete the initial questionnaires, and 26 were lost to follow-up. Despite the dropouts the final sample was generally representative of women who had delivered at the hospital over a 5-year period.

Assessment Measures

Depression and Social Adjustment

The Beck Depression Inventory, or BDI (Beck et al., 1961), was used as the primary measure of depression severity during pregnancy and the puerperium. Level of social adjustment during pregnancy was also assessed (as a predictor of postpartum depression) using the self-report version of the Social Adjustment Scale, or SAS (Weissman & Bothwell, 1976). This instrument contains 54 items assessing role functioning in 5 areas: work, social and leisure, extended family, marital–parental, and family unit.

A subset of the subjects selected on the basis of the postpartum BDI (see the later section entitled "Procedure") participated in a semistructured interview based on the Schedule for Affective Disorders and Schizophrenia, or SADS (Endicott & Spitzer, 1978; O'Hara et al., 1983). The SADS was developed to allow for reliable assessments of the Research Diagnostic Criteria (a forerunner of DSM-III) for depression (Spitzer et al., 1978).

Cognitive–Behavioral Constructs

Four questionnaires were selected to measure constructs relevant to the behavioral, self-control, cognitive, and learned helplessness models of depression. The Interpersonal Events Schedule, or IES (Youngren & Lewinsohn, 1980), was used as a measure of social reinforcement (skill in eliciting social reinforcers). The schedule contains 2 scales assessing the frequency and impact of 70 interpersonal activities and cognitions concerning interpersonal activities (from the original 160 items of the measure). The Self-Control Questionnaire, or SCQ (Rehm et al., 1981), is a 41-item instrument that presents beliefs or attitudes that people have regarding self-control behaviors. Subjects respond on a 7-point Likert-type scale indicating their agreement with each item (e.g., "I am aware of my accomplishments each day"). The Dysfunctional Attitude Scale, or DAS (Weissman & Beck, 1978), is a 40-item instrument, similar in format to the SCQ, designed to assess cognitive distortions. The Attributional Style Questionnaire, or ASQ (Seligman, Abramson, Semmel, & von Baeyer, 1979), was designed to measure attribution constructs relevant to the reformulated learned helplessness model.

Stressful Life Events

The Social Readjustment Rating Scale, or SRRS (Holmes & Rahe, 1967), was used to determine occurrence of stressful life events from the beginning of pregnancy through the postpartum period. A 3-point rating scale of delivery stress was adapted from the delivery record at the hospital where all babies were delivered.

Social Support and Network

For the subset of subjects who participated in the SADS interview, information was obtained regarding the size of the participants' social networks and the total number of confidants available to each participant.

In addition, questions regarding the giving and receiving of instrumental (e.g., babysitting, helping with household tasks) and emotional support were asked regarding the participants' partners, confidants, and parents (O'Hara et al., 1983).

Procedure

Subjects were recruited during a prenatal visit. Each woman's informed consent was obtained; and questionnaires assessing personal history, cognitive–behavioral constructs, and other measures were completed and returned by mail. A delivery stress rating was made from the birth records of each subject. Follow-up depression assessments were conducted, on the average, 11.7 weeks postpartum (ranging from 5.6 to 20.1 weeks). The follow-up assessments with the BDI and the SRRS were conducted over the phone by a trained staff person. A subsample of 42 women who had either high (BDI > 12) or low (BDI < 10) postpartum depression scores were interviewed to establish the presence of a postpartum depression based on RDC (Spitzer et al., 1978). These women also participated in an assessment of the structure and quality of their social networks.

Results

The level of depressive symptomatology did not increase after delivery; rather, it decreased significantly (Pre-BDI Mean = 8.79, SD = 5.91; and Post-BDI Mean = 7.42, SD = 5.23), $t(167) = 3.34$, $p < .01$. Breaking down the BDI into its cognitive–affective items (1–14) and its somatic items (15–21) showed that only the level of the somatic items decreased significantly after delivery. These findings suggested that, at least for level of depressive symptomatology, there is no increase in depression after delivery.

A hierarchical multiple regression was conducted to test the principal hypotheses that prenatal measures of cognitive–behavioral constructs and measures of social adjustment and life stress would account for significant amounts of variance in postpartum depressive symptomatology. Four groups of variables were entered into the regression in the following order: (1) prepartum BDI; (2) measures of cognitive–behavioral constructs; (3) Social Adjustment Scale—self-report; and (4) life stress measures. The overall regression predicting postpartum depression level as measured by the BDI was significant; and each of the groups of variables, with the exception of the social adjustment group, accounted for significant variance in level of postpartum depressive symptomatology (see Table 2.1). Only the measure of attributional style among the cognitive–behavioral measures was significant in the regression. Interestingly, with respect to the stress measures, delivery stress was inversely

TABLE 2.1. Hierarchical multiple regression of psychological and life stress variables on postpartum depression level.

Predictor variable	r	R	ΔR^2	Standardized β	F
Prepartum Beck Depression Inventory	.509***	.509	.259	.509	53.02***
Cognitive–behavioral		.549	.042		2.54*
Dysfunctional Attitude Scale	−.283***	.519	.010	−.063	<1
Attributional Style Questionnaire (composite)	−.304***	.540	.023	−.160	4.54*
Interpersonal Events Schedule (cross product)	−.251**	.541	.001	.071	<1
Self-Control Questionnaire	.313***	.549	.008	.106	1.70
Social Adjustment Scale	.442***	.554	.006	.129	1.37
Life stress		.634	.094		11.38***
Delivery Stress Rating	−.131*	.577	.027	−.155	5.67**
Social Readjustment Rating Scale	.372***	.634	.067	.278	16.43***

*$p < .05$
**$p < .01$
***$p < .001$

Note: $F(8, 145) = 12.15$, $p < .001$. For all of the tests, with 2 exceptions, $df = 1, 145$. For the entire set of cognitive–behavioral variables, $df = 4, 145$, and for the entire set of life stress variables, $df = 2, 145$. From "Predicting depressive symptomatology: Cognitive–behavioral models and postpartum depression" by M.W. O'Hara, L.P. Rehm, & S.B. Campbell, 1982, *Journal of Abnormal Psychology, 91,* 457–461. Copyright 1982 by the American Psychological Association. Reprinted by permission of the publisher.

related to level of postpartum depressive symptomatology. That is, women with less stressful deliveries had higher postpartum depression scores.

From the total sample of 170 subjects, 2 subgroups were selected to participate in a diagnostic interview. Of the 23 who were selected on the basis of low postpartum BDI scores (BDI < 10), 19 subjects were found not to have experienced a major or minor depression during the postpartum period. Conversely, of the 19 women who were selected on the basis of high postpartum BDI scores (BDI > 12), 11 women were found to have experienced a major or minor postpartum depression. These 11 depressed and 19 nondepressed subjects were compared on a number of measures of social support and social network characteristics.

There were no differences between depressed and nondepressed subjects with respect to social network size or total number of confidants (see Table 2.2). However, depressed subjects were more likely than nondepressed subjects to have at least weekly contact with members of their social networks, $\chi^2(1) = 8.20$, $p < .01$.

Partners of depressed subjects were viewed as less able providers of social support. Depressed subjects rated themselves as having more frequent marital problems, $t(27) = 2.46$, $p < .05$, and being less happy in their marriages, $t(27) = -2.20$, $p < .05$. Depressed subjects also reported

TABLE 2.2. Social network size at prenatal and postnatal assessments.

	Postpartum depressed (*N* = 11)		Postpartum nondepressed (*N* = 19)	
Measure	Mean	*SD*	Mean	*SD*
Prenatal self-report: Total network size	10.36	6.20	11.58	7.64
Prenatal self-report: Number of confidants	6.27	4.20	8.37	4.14
Postnatal interview: Total network size	16.91	3.62	18.37	5.22
Postnatal interview: Number of confidants	7.45	3.59	7.26	4.00

Note: Subjects did not differ significantly on any of these measures. From "Postpartum depression: A role for social network and life stress variables" by M.W. O'Hara, L.P. Rehm, & S.B. Campbell, 1983, *Journal of Nervous and Mental Disease, 171,* 336–341.

being less able to rely on their partners for emotional support, $t(27) = +2.27$, $p < .05$, and instrumental support, $t(27) = +3.37$, $p < .01$. Depressed subjects were also less likely to talk over problems with their partners, $t(26) = 2.22$, $p < .05$. Finally, the depressed subjects, $t(9) = 2.54$, $p < .05$, but not the nondepressed subjects, showed a significant drop in marital satisfaction from the prepartum to postpartum assessments.

With respect to confidants and parents, the depressed subjects reported that they were less able to rely on their confidants for emotional support, $t(27) = -2.49$, $p < .05$, and that their confidants were less available to them, $t(27) = 2.64$, $p < .05$. Depressed subjects also reported that they received less emotional support from their mothers, $t(26) = -2.18$, $p < .05$.

Implications

The results of this first study in our series had several important implications. First, there was little evidence that, on the average, women experienced increased levels of depressive symptomatology after delivery relative to pregnancy. Somatic symptoms showed a significant decline after delivery; cognitive symptoms showed no change. Although we demonstrated that levels of depressive symptomatology did not increase after delivery, we were unable to determine whether the rate of clinically significant depression may have increased after delivery. Nor were we able to address the question of the extent to which levels of depressive symptomatology, either before or after delivery, would have differed from nonchildbearing women followed over a similar period. Both of these questions were addressed in studies that will be described later.

Our model of postpartum depression causal factors accounted for 40% of the variance in postpartum depressive symptomatology scores. More than 25% of the variance in postpartum BDI scores was accounted for by the prepartum BDI alone. These findings suggest that there was a high degree of stability in level of depressive symptomatology over a long period during which many life changes were occurring. As a consequence, women who are doing poorly during pregnancy should be carefully watched after delivery because it is likely that their adjustment will be similarly poor.

Despite the high degree of depression stability, the group of cognitive–behavioral variables accounted for a significant portion of additional variance (4.2%) in postpartum depression level. The measure of attributional style was the one measure in this group that achieved statistical significance. Women who during pregnancy attributed negative events (e.g., a failure) to factors that were stable over time, that had widespread significance for their lives, and that were internal to them were at increased risk for elevated levels of postpartum depressive symptomatology. These findings suggest that the way a woman views the world during pregnancy will have implications for her adjustment after delivery.

The two life stress measures accounted for an additional 9.4% of the variance in level of postpartum depressive symptomatology. As expected, higher levels of stressful life events during pregnancy and the early postpartum period were associated with higher levels of postpartum depressive symptomatology. Although it is often difficult to prevent stressful events from occurring, potentially stressful events can sometimes be avoided or delayed (e.g., moving, having an in-law move in, changing jobs). Advice to reduce unnecessary stressors during pregnancy, particularly after delivery, might have a salutary effect for many women (Gordon & Gordon, 1960).

Quite contrary to our expectation was the finding that more stressful deliveries were associated with lower levels of postpartum depressive symptomatology. Although surprising, other studies had obtained similar results (Blumberg, 1980; Paykel et al., 1980). It may be that women with more stressful deliveries receive more social support from their spouses, which reduces the probability of depressive symptomatology (O'Hara et al., 1982).

The analyses involving the clinically depressed and nondepressed postpartum subjects clearly indicated that the depressed women experienced a relative lack of social support from important members of their networks, spouses, confidants, and mothers. These findings, together with the finding that depressed women had a greater amount of contact in the postpartum period with network members, suggest that the women were seeking support from network members but not receiving it. Most of the dissatisfaction expressed by the depressed women was related to their spouses and, to a lesser extent, their confidants. It is clear that the marital relationship and support of the spouse are of vital importance during the postpartum period. The birth of the child (particularly the first one) may represent the fulfillment of the woman's vision regarding her family. Stress in the marital relationship may threaten that vision and cause the woman to reconsider, in a very negative way, her future. Of course, problems in the marital relationship may stem from the husband's uncertainty or ambivalence about his new role more than from any disinterest in or hostility toward the marriage. These findings suggest that a part of childbirth preparation should include attention to the couple's relationship and the changes that it might undergo after delivery.

Postpartum Depression II: Prevalence, Course, and Predictive Factors

The first study in our series left a number of questions unanswered. For example, because we completed only diagnostic interviews with a subsample of our subjects, the rate of diagnostically defined postpartum depression was impossible to ascertain. Up to the time of our second study, there had been virtually no studies of postpartum depression using conventionally defined diagnostic criteria to determine the prevalence of depression (O'Hara & Zekoski, 1988). In order to determine the significance of a given prevalence rate for postpartum depression, it was important to use standard diagnostic criteria (e.g., DSM-III, RDC).

A limited range of predictor variables was evaluated in the regression model of the first study. We sought to expand and improve our predictor variables in the second study, particularly in the areas of depression history and life events. In this study we included assessments of past history of major depression, depression in first-degree relatives, and presence of major or minor depression during pregnancy. With respect to life events, we used a much more adequate measure of stressful life events (Pilkonis, Imber, & Rubinsky, 1985) than had been used in the first study. We also developed a measure of stressful peripartum events that systematically assessed obstetrically related stressors during pregnancy, labor, and delivery (O'Hara, Varner, & Johnson, 1986). Finally, we added a measure of childcare-related stressors occurring during the early postpartum period (Cutrona, 1983).

In the first study, the model was tested only in the context of level of depressive symptomatology as an outcome. In this study, as already described, we assessed depression using the RDC at 2 points in time: during the second trimester of pregnancy and approximately 9-weeks postpartum. As a consequence, we were able to test our predictive model with respect both to level of postpartum depressive symptomatology and diagnostically defined postpartum depression.

Subjects

A total of 99 women were followed from the second trimester of pregnancy through 9 weeks postpartum. They were recruited from one public obstetrics and gynecology clinic and two private practices. Women were eligible for participation if they were married and at least 18 years of age. They had a mean age of 26.5 years, a mean education level of 15.1 grades, and mean length of marriage of 4.1 years. Ninety-eight percent of the sample were Caucasian; 50% were nulliparous.

Assessment Measures

The Beck Depression Inventory was used again as the measure of depressive symptomatology. Depression diagnoses were made in the context of a semistructured interview derived from the Schedule for Affective Disorders and Schizophrenia (Endicott & Spitzer, 1978). Diagnoses of major and minor depression and past history of depression were based on the Research Diagnostic Criteria (Spitzer et al., 1978). Subjects were also asked about first-degree relatives who might have experienced an episode of depression.

The Self-Control Questionnaire and the Attributional Style Questionnaire were used again in this study as indices of cognitive vulnerability to depression. The life stress measures included the Pilkonis Life Events Schedule, or PLES (Pilkonis et al., 1985), the Childcare Stress Inventory, or CSI (Cutrona, 1983), and the Peripartum Events Scale, or PES (O'Hara et al., 1986). These measures assessed, respectively, stressful life events, childcare-related stressors in the early postpartum period, and the stressfulness of labor and delivery. A full description of the SCQ and the life stress measures is found in chapter 3.

Social support was assessed using the Social Support Interview, which was a slightly modified version of the Social Network Interview used in the first study. In this study we focused on the social support provided by the spouse and the woman's closest confidant. We also used the Postpartum Social Support Questionnaire, or PSSQ (Hopkins, Campbell, & Marcus, 1987) to assess social support provided by several groups of individuals, including the woman's spouse, parents, in-laws, other relatives, and friends. Finally, the Dyadic Adjustment Scale, or DAS (Spanier, 1976), was used to assess the quality of the marital relationship. A full description of these measures is found in chapter 3.

Procedure

Subjects were recruited at a prenatal visit during the second trimester. They completed the self-report measures at home and returned for an initial diagnostic interview. The occurrences of major or minor depression during and before pregnancy and depression in family members were determined at this interview. In addition, social support provided by spouses and confidants and the occurrence of stressful life events since the beginning of pregnancy were assessed. In the third trimester of pregnancy and again at 3, 6, and 9 weeks and at 6 months postpartum, self-report assessments of depression and marital adjustment were completed. The follow-up diagnostic interview was completed approximately 9 weeks after delivery. Depression occurring after the initial interview, social support from the spouse and confidant, and stressful life events occurring since the initial interview were determined at this time.

Results

A total of 9 women (9%) experienced either a major or minor depression during pregnancy, and 12 women (12%) experienced a major or minor depression within 9 weeks after delivery. Two women were depressed during pregnancy and after delivery; they both reported that their symptoms were exacerbated after delivery. One-half of the women reported episodes beginning within 1 week of delivery; however, some episodes began as late as 6 weeks postpartum. The mean duration of postpartum episodes was 3.3 weeks (ranging from 1 to 6 weeks).

Similar to the results of the first study, BDI scores were at their highest in the second trimester of pregnancy and declined steadily through 6-months postpartum (see Figure 2.1). Both the somatic and cognitive–affective subscales showed the same pattern.

In these analyses we addressed several questions regarding the relationships between a number of predictor variables and prepartum and

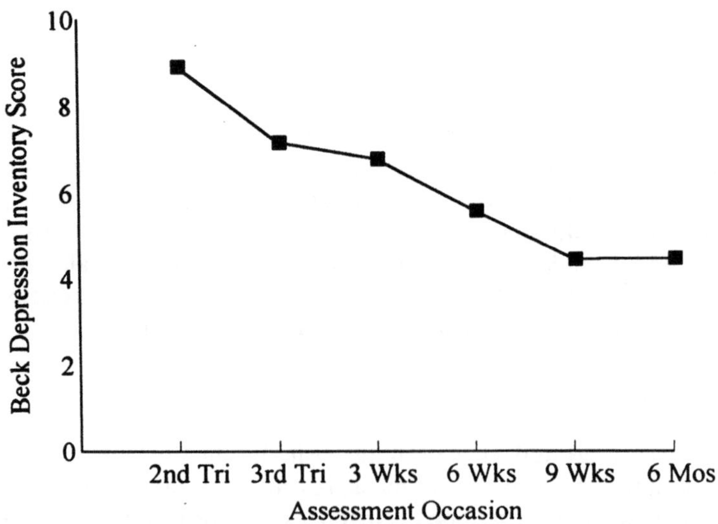

FIGURE 2.1. Beck Depression Inventory scores for women during pregnancy and after delivery. (2nd Tri = second trimester of pregnancy; 3rd Tri = third trimester; 3 Wks = 3 weeks postpartum; 6 Wks = 6 weeks postpartum; 9 Wks = 9 weeks postpartum; 6 Mos = months postpartum.)

postpartum depression. In the first series of analyses, we compared prepartum-depressed and -nondepressed subjects and postpartum-depressed and -nondepressed subjects on variables reflecting sociodemographic status, personal and family history of depression, stressful life events, and social support. The second series of analyses involved testing the vulnerability–life stress model of postpartum depression using hierarchical multiple regression.

With respect to sociodemographic variables, women who experienced depression during pregnancy had more children than women who did not experience depression during pregnancy, $t(97) = -2.01$, $p < .05$. Also, women who experienced a postpartum depression had a lower education level than nondepressed women, $t(97) = 2.21$, $p < .05$. No other sociodemographic variables differentiated the depressed and nondepressed groups (e.g., age, years of marriage, parity).

Previous history of depression and depression in a first-degree relative did not differentiate the prepartum-depressed and -nondepressed subjects. However, postpartum-depressed women had a greater likelihood of having a depressed first-degree relative, $\chi^2(1; N = 99) = 9.26$, $p < .01$, than nondepressed women.

There was no difference between depressed and nondepressed women during pregnancy on the number of stressful life events that occurred between the beginning of pregnancy and the second-trimester interview. Postpartum-depressed women relative to -nondepressed women experienced significantly more stressful life events between delivery and the 9-week postpartum interview, $t(97) = -4.80$, $p < .001$, and significantly more childcare-related stressors during the postpartum period, $t(97) = -2.77$, $p < .01$. There were no differences between postpartum-depressed and -nondepressed subjects with respect to the number of peripartum events (obstetrical stressors).

We also tested the prediction that women experiencing either prepartum or postpartum depression would receive less social support from their spouses and closest confidants than nondepressed women. Women experiencing depression during pregnancy reported receiving less instrumental support from their spouses than did nondepressed women, $t(97) = 3.10$, p 1 $< .01$. Prepartum-depressed women also reported that their spouses were less available when needed, $t(97) = 2.85$, $p < .01$, and made their life less easy, $t(97) = 2.53$, $p < .05$. Interestingly, prepartum-depressed subjects reported being more able to turn to their confidants for emotional support, $t(89) = -2.05$, $p < .05$, and being more likely to talk over problems or troubles with their confidants, $t(89) = -3.58$, $p < .01$.

Postpartum-depressed women reported that they received both less instrumental support, $t(97) = 2.27$, $p < .05$, and emotional support, $t(97) = 2.85$, $p < .01$, from their spouses. Postpartum-depressed women also said that they felt less free to talk about anything they wished with their spouses, $t(97) = 2.76$, $p < .01$, and that their spouses were less available when needed, $t(97) = 2.98$, $p < .01$. Finally, postpartum-depressed women said that they were less able to rely on their spouses for childcare help, $t(97) = 4.14$, $p < .001$, and that their spouses made their lives less easy, $t(97) = 2.35$, $p < .05$. Postpartum-depressed women also reported significantly less marital satisfaction both during pregnancy, $t(97) = 2.59$, $p < .05$, and after delivery, $t(96) = 2.01$, $p < .05$.

The results from the Postpartum Social Support Questionnaire indicated that postpartum-depressed women were dissatisfied with the frequency of supportive behaviors from social-network members. Postpartum-

TABLE 2.3. Hierarchical multiple regression of postpartum depression level on demographic, vulnerability, and life stress factors.

Predictor variable	r	R	ΔR^2	R^2	Standardized β	F
Sociodemographic		.236	.056	.056		1.37
Socioeconomic status	−.092	.092	.008		−.029	
Working during pregnancy	−.098	.130	.009		−.109	
Years of marriage	−.173	.215	.029		−.117	
Age	−.198	.236	.009		−.138	
Depression history		.514	.208	.264		6.29****
Number of previous episodes of depression	.057	.239	.001		.069	<1.00
Depressed first-degree relative	.044	.245	.003		.096	1.01
Depressed during pregnancy	.095	.251	.003		−.189	3.08
Second-trimester Beck Depression Inventory	.458	.514	.201		.562	24.27****
Life stress		.674	.191	.454		10.01****
Pilkonis Life Events Scale	.204	.526	.013		.102	1.41
Obstetric risk factors	.436	.618	.105		.322	14.07****
Childcare stress scale	.425	.674	.072		.302	11.33***
Cognitive		.699	.036	.489		2.88*
Attributional Style Questionnaire	.014	.675	.001		−.080	<1.00
Self-Control Questionnaire	.321	.699	.034		.234	5.54**

*$p = .062$
**$p < .05$
***$p < .01$
****$p < .001$

Notes: $F(13, 84) = 6.19$, $p < .001$. For individual tests, $df = 1, 84$. For socio-demographic and depression history sets, $df = 4, 84$. For life-stress set, $df = 3, 84$. For cognitive set, $df = 2, 84$. From "A prospective study of postpartum depression: Prevalence, course, and predictive factors" by M.W. O'Hara, D.J. Neunaber, & E.M. Zekoski, 1984, *Journal of Abnormal Psychology, 93,* 158–171. Copyright 1984 by the American Psychological Association. Adapted by permission of the publisher.

depressed women expressed dissatisfaction with the frequency of their spouses' supportive behaviors, $t(96) = -2.67$, $p < .01$, and similar dissatisfaction with their parents, $t(96) = -2.93$, $p < .01$, and their parents-in-law, $t(95) = -3.18$, $p < .01$.

Our second major set of analyses involved testing what we called the vulnerability–life stress model of postpartum depression using hierarchical multiple regression. We tested the model in the context of predicting both level of postpartum depressive symptomatology and postpartum diagnostic status. Four major groups of variables were entered into the regression analyses: (1) sociodemographic; (2) depression history; (3) life stress; and (4) cognitive. Tables 2.3 and 2.4 reveal that the

TABLE 2.4. Hierarchical multiple regression of postpartum depression diagnostic status on demographic, vulnerability, and life stress factors.

Predictor variable	r	R	ΔR^2	R^2	Standardized β	F
Sociodemographic		.278	.077	.077		1.95
Socioeconomic status	−.121	.121	.014		−.067	
Working during pregnancy	−.223	.248	.047		−.187	
Years of marriage	.055	.255	.004		.144	
Age	−.124	.278	.012		−.161	
Depression history		.470	.143	.221		4.10**
Number of previous depressions	.250	.363	.055		.172	3.03
Depressed first-degree relative	.340	.470	.088		.314	10.04***
Depressed during pregnancy	.097	.470	.000		−.020	<1.00
Second-trimester Beck Depression Inventory	.075	.470	.000		.023	<1.00
Life stress		.558	.090	.311		3.74*
Pilkonis Life Events Scale	.245	.516	.045		.200	4.26*
Obstetric risk factors	−.034	.516	.000		−.003	<1.00
Childcare stress scale	.269	.558	.044		.237	5.53*
Cognitive		.560	.003	.314		<1.00
Attributional Style Questionnaire	.038	.559	.002		.054	
Self-Control Questionnaire	−.054	.560	.001		−.039	

*$p = .05$
**$p < .01$
***$p < .001$

Notes: $F(13, 84) = 2.95$, $p < .01$. For individual tests, $df = 1, 84$. For sociodemographic and depression history sets, $df = 4, 84$. For life stress set, $df = 3, 84$. For cognitive set, $df = 2, 84$. From "A prospective study of postpartum depression: Prevalence, course, and predictive factors" by M.W. O'Hara, D.J. Neunaber, & E.M. Zekoski, 1984, *Journal of Abnormal Psychology, 93,* 158–171. Copyright 1984 by the American Psychological Association. Adapted by permission of the publisher.

patterns of results for the two outcome measures were different. The major variables accounting for significant variance in level of postpartum depressive symptomatology were level of prepartum depressive symptomatology from the depression history group, level of obstetric risk factors and childcare stress from the life stress group, and self-control beliefs from the cognitive group. With respect to postpartum depression diagnostic status, the major predictors were depressed first-degree relative from the depression history group, stressful life events since the beginning of pregnancy, and level of childcare stressors from the life stress group. Altogether, the variables in our model accounted for almost 50% of the variance in postpartum depressive symptomatology but only 31% of the variance in postpartum diagnostic status.

Implications

Although the rate of postpartum depression appeared to be high (i.e., 12%) and it was one-third higher than during pregnancy (9%), the difference was not significant. These rates were similar to those reported by other investigators in both Great Britain and the United States (Cutrona, 1983; Kumar & Robson, 1984; Watson et al., 1984). At issue was the question of whether these depression rates exceeded those of nonchildbearing women. The initial results from the NIMH Epidemiological Catchment Area (ECA) study (Myers et al., 1984) indicated that the 6-month–period prevalence of major depression in women ages 18 to 44 was between 3.0% and 7.4%. The criteria, used in the ECA study were more stringent than our criteria, but they reflect depression over a period (6 months) that was 3 times longer than the postpartum period that we studied (roughly 2 months). The ambiguity of our findings regarding the extent to which the postpartum period represented a "high-risk" time for depression pointed to the importance of a controlled prospective study of postpartum depression to begin to resolve this issue.

Similar to the results of our earlier study and in spite of the fact that the prevalence of depression was higher after delivery than during pregnancy, level of depressive symptomatology declined from the second trimester through 9 weeks and 6-months postpartum. This effect was particularly marked for the somatic relative to the cognitive symptoms of depression. In nonchildbearing women the ratio of level of somatic to cognitive symptoms was much lower than what we found for the childbearing women (O'Hara et al., 1984). These findings suggest that part of the elevation in scores on measures like the Beck Depression Inventory during pregnancy and the early postpartum period is due to the normal physiological changes that accompany childbearing. These findings also point to the importance of taking into account these normal physiological changes when assessing depression by means of interview or self-report.

This study yielded several important risk factors for diagnostically defined postpartum depression. Women who had a depressed first-degree relative or experienced stressful life events were at increased risk for diagnostically defined postpartum depression. These findings fit very well with our understanding that depression tends to run in families (Mendlewicz, 1985) and that its risk is increased by stressful life events (Brown & Harris, 1978). They also suggest the importance of cross-fertilization between depression research with childbearing and nonchildbearing women. The processes may be very similar, if not identical.

Women who had elevated levels of depressive symptomatology during pregnancy, who had relatively more dysfunctional self-control attitudes, or who experienced higher levels of obstetrical risk factors and stressful events related to childcare were at increased risk for elevated levels of depressive symptomatology after delivery. These findings were consistent with results of our earlier study and suggest that the negative affect reflected in the BDI is very stable and is tied to more dysfunctional thinking and negative life events than to a personal and family history of clinical depression. Further implications of these findings will be developed in chapters 8 and 9.

There was little overlap among the prepartum- and postpartum-depressed women. Moreover, there were important differences between women experiencing prepartum versus postpartum depression with respect to the variables associated with depression during the prepartum and postpartum periods. For example, women experiencing prepartum depression, unlike women experiencing postpartum depression, did not differ from nondepressed subjects on the number of stressful life events that they had experienced, their level of marital satisfaction, or their personal and family histories of depression. Also, their complaints about lack of support from spouses were not as broad.

What might have accounted for the observed differences in factors associated with prepartum and postpartum depression? As already suggested, the pattern of results for postpartum depression was in accord with earlier literature related to both postpartum depression and depression occurring at other times (Brown & Harris, 1978; O'Hara et al., 1984; Paykel et al., 1980). The results for depression during pregnancy did not follow the expected pattern. One possible explanation is that physical distress (i.e., somatic discomfort) may have been more responsible for depressions occurring during pregnancy than for depressions occurring during the puerperium. That is, some of the prepartum-depressed women may have been significantly bothered by somatic disturbance during pregnancy. We found that somatic symptoms relative to cognitive–affective symptoms are highest during pregnancy and immediately after delivery and then drop throughout the postpartum period. Also, women who were depressed during pregnancy had significantly more children than nondepressed women and may have been unable to rest when they felt ill. Paffenbarger (1982) obtained similar findings in a study of severe peripartum illness. Although these data are not definitive, they do suggest that it may be worthwhile to monitor carefully the extent to which physical discomfort affects mood during pregnancy to determine if there is a link between somatic disturbance and depression during this period.

Postpartum Depression II: $4\frac{1}{2}$-Year Follow-Up of Women and Children

Postpartum depression exists within a family context. Our work had suggested that whether a cause or a consequence, there were significant disturbances in the marital relationships of postpartum-depressed women. Because depression is a recurrent and sometimes chronic disorder, many women who experience postpartum depression will have recurrences of depression. However, the evidence with respect to future risk for depression (over a 3- to 5-year period) for women who have experienced a postpartum depression has been somewhat mixed (Kumar & Robson, 1984; Wolkind et al., 1980; Wrate 1985; et al., 1985; Uddenberg & Englesson, 1978). We hoped to clarify the risk for future depression in the first American sample of depressed and nondepressed childbearing women to be followed over a period of several years.

Postpartum depression may also have significant consequences for the child. For example, postpartum depression might be expected to disrupt the development of the mother–child relationship and have deleterious consequences for the child's development. Children of depressed women appear to be at risk for a variety of cognitive and behavioral problems (Hammen, 1991). These negative consequences are apparent in infants, toddlers, and school-age children (Cytryn et al., 1984; Gaensbauer, Harmon, Cytryn, & McKnew, 1984; Weintraub, Neale, & Liebert, 1975; Zahn-Waxler, McKnew, Cummings, Davenport, & Radke-Yarrow, 1984). Moreover, results of investigations of depressed mothers and young infants indicate that mother–child interactions are negative relative to nondepressed mother–infant dyads (Cohn et al., 1990; Field, Healy, Goldstein, & Guthertz, 1990).

The findings with respect to the long-term consequences of postpartum depression for the child have been mixed. Uddenberg and Englesson (1978) found evidence of disturbance in the mother–child relationship based on interviews with both mothers and children at a $4\frac{1}{2}$-year follow-up. Ghodsian et al. (1984) found that children of postpartum-depressed mothers who were followed up at 42 months of age were reported to have more behavioral problems than children of mothers who did not experience a postpartum depression. Using the same measure of child behavior problems as Ghodsian et al., Wrate et al., (1985) found that briefer postpartum depressions (compared to no depression and lengthy postpartum depressions) were associated with higher levels of child behavior problems at a 3-year follow-up. Finally, the only follow-up study in which there was direct assessment of child function found that children of postpartum-depressed women had significantly lower scores on the McCarthy Scales of Children's Abilities, a test of a variety of aspects of cognitive performance (Cogill et al., 1986). However, these investigators found no relation between postpartum depression and later child social and emotional problems (Caplan et al., 1989). The interpretation of the findings in these studies is complicated by the fact that child adjustment problems at follow-up were also associated with maternal depression at follow-up, making it difficult to attribute increased child behavior problems specifically to the women's earlier postpartum depression (Ghodsian et al., 1984).

These considerations persuaded us to follow up the women and their children born at the time of their participation in our earlier study (O'Hara et al., 1984; Philipps & O'Hara, 1991). We determined whether the participants experienced any depressive episodes during the $4\frac{1}{2}$-year follow-up period, and we assessed the psychosocial adjustment of the participants at the time of the follow-up interview. We assessed child behavior problems using the internalizing and externalizing scales of the Child Behavior Checklist (Achenbach & Edelbrock, 1983). We expected that women who had experienced a postpartum depression would be more likely to experience a depressive episode during the $4\frac{1}{2}$-year follow-up period and would report a higher level of internalizing and externalizing problems in their children than women who did not experience a postpartum depression.

Subjects

Subjects were 70 of 99 women who participated in our earlier study (O'Hara et al., 1984). Women who completed the current study had a mean age of 31.4 years (SD = 3.8), a mean education level of 15.7 years (SD = 2.3), and 47% were employed. They had an average of 2 children, and 53% of the subjects had at least 1 child subsequent to their participation in the original study. All but 1 of the subjects were Caucasian. At follow-up, 91.5% of the women were married, 8.5% were separated or divorced, and 1.4% had been divorced and remarried.

Measures

All depression diagnoses were made in the context of our semistructured interview adapted from the SADS (Endicott & Spitzer, 1978). Major and minor depressions that occurred anytime during the $4\frac{1}{2}$-year follow-up and depressive episodes at the time of the follow-up interview were diagnosed according to the RDC (Spitzer et al., 1978). The BDI was used once again as our measure of depressive symptomatology.

Children's behavior was assessed through mothers' reports using the Child Behavior Checklist, or CBCL (Achenbach & Edelbrock, 1983). The CBCL consists of 118 behavioral items what assess difficulties a child may exhibit, reflecting phenomena such as depression, withdrawal, hyperactivity, and aggression. A parent is asked to rate her child's behavior during the previous 6 months on a 3-point scale: 0 = "not true," 1 = "somewhat or sometimes true," and 2 = "very true or often true." There is good evidence for the reliability and validity of the CBCL (Achenbach, 1978; Achenbach & Edelbrock, 1979; Cohen, Gotlieb, Kershner, & Wehrspann, 1985).

Procedure

Subjects were recruited by a letter that was sent to their last known address. If a subject had moved, attempts were made to contact her through forwarding addresses as well as through relatives and friends whose names had been provided in the original study. The letter was followed up by a phone call. The study was described to each subject, and her informed consent was obtained. Subjects who agreed to participate received the BDI, CBCL, and other measures to complete at home and return by mail. Of those subjects whom we were unable to follow up successfully, 5 agreed to participate initially but did not complete the study, 7 declined to participate, and we were unable to locate the remaining 17 women.

Subjects completed a diagnostic interview with an interviewer blind to their status in the original study within approximately 14 days of completing their questionnaires. Women residing in the local area (within a 40-mile radius—roughly one-third of the sample) were interviewed in their homes or in our laboratory. Women residing outside of the local area were interviewed over the phone. During the interview information concerning demographics and depression occurring during the $4\frac{1}{2}$-year follow-up period was obtained.

Results

There were no differences between the subjects who participated in the follow-up investigation and those who did not with respect to demographic characteristics and depression (based on the original investigation). Moreover, 10 of the 12 women who had experienced a postpartum depression during the original investigation participated in the follow-up study.

Four women (5.7%) were diagnosed as experiencing a minor or major depression at the time of the $4\frac{1}{2}$-year follow-up interview (one of whom had experienced a postpartum depression). A total of 33 women (47.1%) experienced at least 1 major or minor depression during the $4\frac{1}{2}$-year follow-up period prior to the follow-up interview. The mean length of episodes during the follow-up period was 38.6 weeks (SD = 42.0); the median length was 16 weeks.

Of the 10 women in the sample who had experienced a postpartum depression, 8 women (80%) experienced another depression during the follow-up period, as compared to 25 of the 60 women (42%) who had not experienced a postpartum depression. There was a significant association between postpartum depression and depression during the follow-up period $\chi^2(1; N = 70) = 3.63, p < .06$). We also compared the postpartum-depressed and -nondepressed subjects on the length of time between delivery and a first nonpostpartum episode of depression (if one occurred) using survival analysis (Lee, 1980). The median survival time (between delivery and a nonpostpartum depression) for the women who experienced a postpartum depression was 132 weeks; for the women who did not experience a postpartum depression, it was 264 weeks (Lee-Desu = 4.87, $df = 1, p < .05$) (Lee & Desu, 1972). The median survival time for the subjects who had not experienced a postpartum is longer than the actual follow-up period because most of these women had not had an episode of depression by the end of the follow-up.

The mean T-score for the internalizing scale of the Child Behavior Checklist was 49.24 (SD = 8.35), for the externalizing scale, it was 49.34 (SD = 9.00). These scores were very similar to the normative samples for these two scales, which by definition had a mean T-score of 50 and SD of 10 (Achenbach & Edelbrock, 1983), suggesting that, on the whole, the children followed up in this study were fairly representative of $4\frac{1}{2}$-year-old children. However, the diagnosis of postpartum depression was not predictive of scores on the internalizing, $t(68) = -1.00$, n.s., and externalizing, $t(68) < 1.$, n.s., scales of the CBCL. Nevertheless, there was a significant association between maternal depression (RDC-defined) during the follow-up period and scores on the internalizing scale, $t(68) = -2.70, p < .01$, and the externalizing scale, $t(68) = -1.92, p < .05$) at the $4\frac{1}{2}$-year follow-up. This finding did not appear to be influenced by level of maternal depressive symptomatology at the time of the follow-up assessment.

Implications

Women who experienced a postpartum depression were at increased risk for later depressions. This increased risk was evidenced by the significant association between postpartum depression and later depression during the $4\frac{1}{2}$-year follow-up period. The increased risk was also evidenced by the survival analysis, which indicated that the average interval between delivery and a later episode of depression was twice as long for women who did not experience a postpartum depression relative to those who did experience a postpartum depression. These findings are consistent with the findings of some of the European studies that women who experience postpartum depression remain vulnerable to future depression at least for the first several years after childbirth (Uddenberg & Englesson, 1978; Wolkind et al., 1980).

In contrast to the results of several follow-up studies (e.g., Ghodsian et al., 1984; Uddenberg & Englesson, 1978), we found no evidence of a direct association between postpartum depression and child behavior problems. However, postpartum depression was associated with increased risk for depression during the follow-up period, which in turn was associated with higher scores on the CBCL. As illustrated in Figure 2.2, postpartum depression may affect child behavior by increasing a woman's risk for later nonpostpartum depressions. Ghodsian et al. (1984) made a similar argument in interpreting the findings from their follow-up study. In our study these later depressions, which occurred closer in time to the child behavior assessments, may be causally related to the higher levels of internalizing and externalizing problems in the $4\frac{1}{2}$-year-old children of the women who had experienced a postpartum depression.

Our earlier work (O'Hara, 1986; O'Hara et al., 1983; O'Hara et al., 1984) and that of others (Campbell et al., 1992; Paykel et al., 1980; Watson et al., 1984) has found that postpartum depression is associated with a past personal and family history of depression. These studies suggest that postpartum depression may be associated with an increased risk for later nonpostpartum depression because it serves as a marker for a general vulnerability to depression. That is, women who have a personal and family history of depression are at increased risk for postpartum

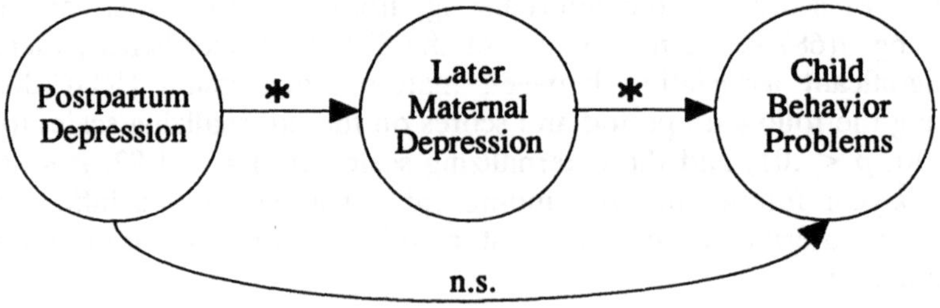

FIGURE 2.2. Model of the relationship between postpartum depression and later child behavior problems (*= path is significant; n.s. = path is not significant). From "Prospective study of postpartum depression: $4\frac{1}{2}$-year follow-up of women and children" by L.H.C. Philipps & M.W. O'Hara, 1991, *Journal of Abnormal Psychology, 100,* 151–155. Copyright 1991 by the American Psychological Association, Inc. Reprinted by permission of the publisher.

depression, which in turn places them at increased risk for later depressions. The later depressions may have deleterious effects on both marital relationships and children.

Looking Forward

Although a great deal was learned about the prevalence, causes, and consequences of postpartum depression, a number of important questions remained to be addressed. For example, Are rates of depression after childbirth elevated relative to times of nonchildbearing? Are risk factors for depression after childbirth and depression that occurs outside of childbearing similar, or are different processes involved? What role do hormonal factors play in postpartum depression? Are the postpartum blues, which we had not previously investigated, related to postpartum depression? Do these two syndromes have similar risk factors? Does the blues lead to depression? A controlled prospective study would be needed to address these questions. The rest of this monograph describes our attempt to answer these questions.

3
Background and Methods

Much of the general background for the study that will be described in this monograph has been presented in chapters 1 and 2. In the first part of this chapter, the background for the specific questions that we addressed will be sketched. These include: (1) What is the prevalence of mood disorders during pregnancy and the puerperium relative to nonchildbearing periods? (2) In what ways do childbearing and nonchildbearing women differ psychologically when followed longitudinally? (3) What factors put women at risk for depression during pregnancy and for the blues and depression after delivery? In the second part of this chapter, the methods that we employed in this study will be outlined.

Increased Risk for Depression in the Postpartum Period

At the time this study was initiated in 1984, there was a great deal of uncertainty in the literature regarding the extent to which the postpartum period was a high-risk time for depression. Several well-done prospective studies using diagnostic criteria to establish the presence of postpartum depression had reported what appeared to be relatively high rates of depression (Kumar & Robson, 1984; Watson et al., 1984). In our own work (O'Hara et al., 1984), as discussed in the last chapter, we found that 12% of our subjects experienced a major or minor depression during the first 9 weeks postpartum. These depressions, with 2 exceptions, all began after delivery; and even in the 2 cases that were exceptions, there was a postpartum exacerbation of the depression. However, there was also a 9% prevalence of depression during the second trimester of pregnancy, suggesting that any increased risk for depression after delivery was not dramatic. In the last chapter it was argued that these pregnancy depressions may have been related to somatic disturbances associated with pregnancy more than to traditional depression risk factors (e.g., stressful life events, prior depression), as was the case for the postpartum depressions. This explanation leaves open the possibility that postpartum depressions may be increased relative to nonchildbearing times if not relative to pregnancy.

In one of the earliest studies using diagnostic criteria to define depression, Cox et al. (1982) found that only 4% of 105 women from Edinburgh, Scotland, had experienced a depressive episode during pregnancy, as compared to 13% who experienced a postpartum depression and were still depressed 3 to 5 months postpartum. Another 16% of subjects were reported to have experienced a milder depression after delivery, which had remitted by the time of the 3- to 5-month postpartum interview.

Cutrona (1983), studying a sample of 85 American women, reported a point prevalence of major depression of 3.5% in the third trimester, as compared to 4.7% two weeks after delivery and 3.5% eight weeks after delivery. This study is notable in that it was the only one to use the DSM-III criteria (APA, 1980) to define depression in a postpartum sample.

Kumar and Robson (1984) followed 119 British women from the first trimester of pregnancy through 1 year postpartum. They found a 10% incidence (new cases) of depression in the first trimester of pregnancy, which was significantly greater than the 1% incidence of depression in the trimester before pregnancy. The incidence of depression dropped to 2.5% in the second and third trimesters of pregnancy and increased to 13.5% in the first 12 weeks after delivery. One woman experienced a continuation of depression from pregnancy to the postpartum period. These findings provided interesting evidence regarding an increased rate of depression associated with both early pregnancy and the early postpartum period, both important periods of reproductive transition.

Watson et al. (1984) conducted a similar study with British women and found that 13% of their 128 subjects experienced a depressive episode during pregnancy and 22% experienced a depressive episode in the first year postpartum; 12% of subjects experienced a depressive episode in the first 6 weeks postpartum. They noted that their 12% period prevalence rate for the first 6 weeks postpartum was similar to a 1-month period prevalence rate of depression among women in the Camberwell section of London (Bebbington, Hurry, Tennant, Sturt, & Wing, 1981).

These studies painted a mixed picture regarding the extent to which the postpartum period is a time of increased risk for depression. One major problem in these studies was the lack of an appropriate comparison group. For example, several of the studies found that rates of depression were greater, though not necessarily significantly greater, after delivery than during pregnancy. Yet it was unclear whether rates of depression during pregnancy were representative of rates of depression at other times in a woman's life. Moreover, the period of time considered during pregnancy for a diagnosis of depression was not always equal to the period of time considered after delivery for a diagnosis of depression. For example, Cox et al. (1982) reported the prevalence of depression for the entire pregnancy (9-month period) and the prevalence of depression after delivery for a 3- to 5-month period. In these cases the rates of depression reported are not directly comparable. A similar problem exists in comparing rates of depression across studies, such as was the case in Watson et al. (1984), because the methods and populations may not be directly comparable. In sum, by the middle of the 1980s, there was some empirical evidence of an increased risk for depression in the postpartum period but data directly comparing rates of depression in childbearing and nonchildbearing samples were still lacking.

Estimates of the prevalence of the postpartum blues have been much more variable than estimates of the prevalence of postpartum depression (O'Hara, 1991). There has never been a question in the postpartum blues literature as to whether its symptoms are common at other times in a woman's life. However, a few investigations have assessed the extent to which symptoms of the blues are common following minor and major nonobstetrical surgical procedures. These studies have found that the blues symptoms are relatively common post surgically in women but their intensity and timing appear to be different from what is observed after delivery. Blues symptoms tend to peak at high levels immediately after a surgical procedure and decline thereafter, whereas blues symptoms after delivery increase to intermediate levels up to about day 5 postpartum and then decline (Kendell et al., 1984; Levy, 1987). Our prospective study provided the first opportunity to assess symptoms of the blues in a nonchildbearing sample of normal women.

The Acquaintance Control Group

The establishment of a proper control group for a prospective study of childbearing women was an important goal of our study (O'Hara, 1989). Because a large majority of women in our community receive prenatal care, recruiting subjects from both public clinics and private practices was thought to result in a sample representative of childbearing women (O'Hara, 1989). However, recruiting nonchildbearing women as controls from public gynecology clinics and private practices was not likely to yield a sample representative of nonchildbearing women. Although most women who receive obstetrical care are healthy, the same is not always the case for women receiving gynecological care. Routine gynecological examinations are becoming more common; however, many women receiving gynecological services are doing so because of illness. As a result, nonchildbearing women receiving gynecological care are probably not representative of nonchildbearing women in general.

Another strategy to recruit a control sample would have been to use some other basis to identify potential controls, such as census data or random sampling from the community as a whole. Assuming that such a strategy were feasible, the control group might differ systematically from the childbearing group on factors such as age, marital status, social class, and parity. This possibility existed because childbearing women are not themselves representative of adult women. For example, they are more likely to be married and to have a restricted age range.

Our solution to these problems was to ask each childbearing subject to nominate five acquaintances who were similar on factors such as age, marital status, working status, and parity. We selected the most similar potential control and invited her to participate in our study. Each control was yoked to her childbearing acquaintance so that she completed the same measures (except the hormonal ones) at the same times as her childbearing acquaintance.

The acquaintance control group has several advantages over other control groups. In addition to being similar to the childbearing women on variables such as age and marital status, the acquaintance controls were likely to be similar on variables such as education, social class, race, community of residence, interests, and other variables that are likely to be similar among acquaintances. Moreover, the acquaintance control group gave us a rational basis for timing assessments in a prospective study. Rather than selecting average or arbitrary times to conduct assessments with controls, we used the timing of assessments of childbearing subjects as the basis for determining the time of assessments of nonchildbearing subjects. In this way the intervals between assessments were equivalent across groups, as were factors such as the season of the year in which assessments were conducted. Also, the use of matched controls provided for increased precision in estimating the association between childbearing and depression (Kelsey, Thompson, & Evans, 1986; Kleinbaum, Kupper, & Morgenstern, 1982; Kupper, Karon, Kleinbaum, Morgenstern, & Lewis, 1981). Finally, because childbearing subjects provided names of potential control subjects, acquaintance controls were much more efficiently recruited than other possible control groups.

The Vulnerability–Life Stress Model of Postpartum Depression

One of the goals of this study was to test the vulnerability–life stress model of postpartum depression. We had tested this model in earlier studies (O'Hara et al., 1982; 1984) and generally had found support for it (see chapter 2). The basic premise of the vulnerability–life stress model is that there are psychological, social, cognitive, and biological forms of vulnerability to depression that interact with environmental stressors to increase a woman's risk for depression (O'Hara, Schlechte, Lewis, & Varner, 1991). One additional assumption for the current study was that this whole process was potentiated by the fact that all subjects were undergoing a demanding and stressful life experience (i.e., childbirth).

The availability of a nonchildbearing control group allowed us to test this assumption.

Depression Vulnerability

Five groups of variables were evaluated in the context of the vulnerability–life stress model: (1) sociodemographic; (2) depression history vulnerability; (3) social and cognitive vulnerability; (4) life stress; and (5) the interaction of the vulnerability and life stress variables. The variables in the sociodemographic group included: (a) socioeconomic status; (b) working during pregnancy; (c) marital status; and (d) age. Overall, sociodemographic factors have shown an uncertain relation to postpartum depression (O'Hara & Zekoski, 1988). For example, O'Hara and Zekoski (1988) reviewed 13 studies that reported on the relationship between SES and postpartum depression (variously defined). Only two studies (Feggetter & Gath, 1981; Playfair & Gowers, 1981) reported a significant association between SES and postpartum depression, both in the predicted direction. Nevertheless, measures of sociodemographic status were included in the model as control variables.

Depression History as an Index of Vulnerability

Depression is a recurrent disorder (Belsher & Costello, 1988), so it is not surprising that women who have experienced depression in the past (i.e., before pregnancy) would be at increased risk for postpartum depression. Interestingly, only a few studies have actually examined this premise in the context of testing a general model of depression or postpartum depression (Lewinsohn, Hoberman, & Rosenbaum, 1988; O'Hara et al., 1984). In our study we were interested in indexing depression history in several ways. First, we indexed depression by conducting a diagnostic interview with all of the women during the second trimester of pregnancy. Women completed a Beck Depression Inventory at the same time to index the level of depressive symptomatology they were experiencing. We also determined whether women met criteria for major depression at any time in their lives prior to their pregnancies; and, if so, we determined how many episodes they had experienced. Finally, we conducted a family history interview to determine whether or not any first-degree family members (i.e., parents and siblings) had ever experienced an episode of depression.

Cognitive and Social Sources of Vulnerability

There are numerous depression theories and measures of theoretical constructs relevant to those theories that could have been selected to serve as the basis for assessing cognitive and social sources of vulnerability in this study. Because of the constraints of assessing variables from a large number of domains, we were not able to employ elaborate measures of cognitive vulnerability (e.g., extensive assessments of depression schema-based cognitive processing). The results of our earlier study (O'Hara et al., 1984), discussed in chapter 2, suggested that the cognitive–behavioral variables were more likely to show an association with levels of postpartum depressive symptomatology than postpartum diagnostic status. This consideration, as well as limitations on the number of variables that could be assessed, led to the decision to measure self-control attitudes (Rehm, 1977) as an index of cognitive vulnerability and to measure marital satisfaction as a measure of social vulnerability (Monroe, Bromet, Connell, & Steiner, 1986). Research on the self-control model of depression has been a long-standing interest of our group (O'Hara et al., 1982; O'Hara et al., 1984). Marital satisfaction is an important variable in its own right, and both prepartum and postpartum marital satisfaction were related to postpartum depression in our previous study (O'Hara, 1986), discussed in chapter 2.

Life Stress

Negative life events have long been recognized as a potential cause of depression (Paykel, 1979). Despite a number of methodological difficulties with life events research (Monroe & Peterman, 1988), studies have consistently found a link between stressful life events and depression, defined both in terms of clinical diagnosis and high symptom levels (Monroe & Peterman, 1988; Paykel, 1982). Stressful life events have been found to be associated with postpartum depression in several studies, including our work (Cutrona, 1983; O'Hara et al., 1983; 1984; Paykel et al., 1980). These events may be especially troublesome during pregnancy and after delivery because the woman is already coping with new burdens. The measure of negative life events that we used, the Pilkonis Life Events Scale (Pilkonis et al., 1985), was designed to assess a wide array of negative life events.

Two more specialized life events measures were also included in this study. In addition to assessing negative life events of the sort that are usually measured in depression research, we sought to measure the potential stressfulness of the medical aspects of pregnancy, labor, and delivery. Events of this sort are rarely found on typical life events measures and are not often spontaneously reported by women. A second domain of particular relevance to this study of postpartum depression was childcare-related stressors. These events are probably more similar to "daily hassles" (DeLongis, Coyne, Dakof, Folkman, & Lazarus, 1982) than to larger, more serious life events; however, in the aggregate they can be very taxing to the woman's coping resources.

Interaction of Depression Vulnerability and Life Stress

The vulnerability–life stress model implies that vulnerability and life stress variables interact to increase a woman's risk for depression after delivery. For the childbearing subjects, there were 18 variables in the vulnerability X life stress group, reflecting the product of 6 variables representing vulnerability to depression and 3 variables representing life stress. For the nonchildbearing subjects, there were 6 variables in the vulnerability X life stress group, reflecting the product of 6 variables representing vulnerability to depression and 1 variable representing life stress. The measures of obstetric stress and early childcare-related stressors were not relevant for the nonchildbearing subjects.

Social Support and Postpartum Depression

In this study we assessed social support provided by the women's partners, parents, and confidants. Our earlier work had indicated that amount and kind of social support provided by spouses and confidants are related to risk for postpartum depression (O'Hara, 1986). Because of these findings and similar findings of other investigators (Cutrona, 1983), we examined the relation between several types and sources of social support and postpartum depression. As we described in the earlier section entitled "Cognitive and Social Sources of Vulnerability", a measure of marital satisfaction was used to represent the construct of social support (from the spouse) when we tested the vulnerability–life stress model of postpartum depression.

Hormonal Etiology of Postpartum Depression

Because of the dramatic changes in hormone levels after delivery, a number of theories have been developed to account for postpartum mood disorders in terms of a relatively unique hormonal dysfunction (Dalton, 1980; George & Sandler, 1988; Stein, 1982; Steiner, 1979). This perspective recognizes that a woman's hormonal milieu undergoes dramatic changes at the time of parturition (George & Sandler, 1988). Levels of hormones such as progesterone, estrogens, and prolactin rise to very high levels by the end of pregnancy and decrease rather abruptly after delivery. A second perspective assumes that hormonal influences on postpartum mood disorders are much the same as they are for mood disorders that occur at other times (O'Hara & Zekoski, 1988). Of particular interest from this perspective are hormones such as cortisol and neurotransmitters such as noradrenaline (Gard et al., 1986; Handley et al., 1980).

One hormonal hypothesis tested in this study was that postpartum-depressed women would experience significantly lower levels of progesterone, estriol, and estradiol and significantly higher levels of prolactin than nondepressed women. It was also predicted that postpartum-depressed women would show significantly higher levels of cortisol after delivery and after a dexamethasone-suppression test administered 3 days after delivery.

Risk Factors for Depression During Pregnancy

Although the principal thrust of the work to be reported in this monograph concerns postpartum adjustment, we were also concerned about the prevalence of and the risk factors for depression during pregnancy. Because the investigation of risk factors for depression during pregnancy was only partially prospective, there were limits to the range of variables that we could evaluate as risk factors and limits to the inferences that we could make based on the largely cross-sectional design of the pregnancy part of the study. Our earlier research had suggested that, relative to depression after delivery, different causal factors may be important in depression during pregnancy. To the extent possible, we evaluated the same risk factors for depression during pregnancy as we did for depression after delivery (O'Hara, 1986).

Methods of Study

Subjects

Subjects were 182 of 191 women who were initially recruited from a public obstetrics and gynecology clinic and 2 private practices at the University of Iowa Hospitals and Clinics. Subjects were eligible for participation if they were at least 18 years of age. Each subject was asked to provide the names of 5 acquaintances who were of similar age, marital and work status, and who had a similar number of children. The acquaintance who appeared most similar to the subject in question was sent a description of the study and asked to participate. If this acquaintance declined, the next most similar acquaintance was contacted. A total of 179 of 189 controls completed the study. Demographic characteristics of the childbearing and nonchildbearing control subjects are displayed in Table 3.1.

Of the 418 pregnant women who were approached, 191 agreed to participate. Reasons for refusal included: (1) not interested (*N* = 79); (2) unwilling to participate in blood draws, 24-hour urine collection, or dexamethasone suppression test (*N* = 36); (3) possible video taping (*N* =

TABLE 3.1. Demographic characteristics of subjects.

Variable	Childbearing subjects	Nonchildbearing controls	t	$\chi^2(N = 177)$	df
Age					175
M	27.02	27.51	−1.41		
SD	4.71	5.04			
Socioeconomic status					175
M	3.71	3.74	−0.52		
SD	1.26	1.07			
Education					176
M	15.18	14.84	1.69		
SD	2.61	2.37			
% working	67.0	74.9		2.44	1
% married	81.9	80.4		<1	1
Years married					137
M	4.41	6.25	−4.63**		
SD	3.09	4.67			
% with 1 or more children	43.3	59.2	−3.54*		176
% private patients	49.5				

*$p < .05$
**$p < .01$
Note: Paired t tests were used. McNemar's chi-square test was used for percentage working and for percentage married. For percentage with 1 or more children, the t test used the actual number of children of childbearing and nonchildbearing subjects. From "Controlled prospective study of postpartum mood disorders: Comparison of childbearing and non-childbearing women" by M.W. O'Hara, E.M. Zekoski, L.H. Philipps, & E.J. Wright, 1990, *Journal of Abnormal Psychology, 99,* 3–15. Copyright 1990 by the American Psychological Association. Reprinted by permission of the publisher.

3); (4) too busy (N = 39); (5) moving, husband reluctant, participation in an earlier study (e.g., O'Hara et al., 1984), no acquaintances for control (N = 64); and (6) anxious about pregnancy (N = 6). Among the women refusing to participate, 88.5% were private patients, 65.2% were working, and 90.3% were married. Their average age was 28.5 years. In general, the refusers were more likely to be married and private patients than were the participants. Private patients are typically women with insurance or personal resources to pay for care by staff physicians. Indigent patients are seen in a clinic staffed by residents who are supervised by staff physicians.

Of the 237 acquaintances who were approached, 189 agreed to participate. Among the 189 women agreeing to participate, 127 were our first choices from the acquaintances lists, 21 were the only acquaintances listed by a childbearing subject, 28 were our second choices, and 11 were our third choices. There were 2 subjects for whom no acquaintances were available, and we selected similar controls from among the acquaintances listed by other childbearing subjects. One childbearing subject withdrew from the study before an acquaintance control could be recruited; and for 1 childbearing subject, no acquaintance control could be recruited.

A total of 9 childbearing subjects dropped out during the study for the following reasons: (1) lost interest/too much work ($N = 3$); (2) moved away ($N = 3$); (3) no control available ($N = 1$); (4) husband decided against continued participation ($N = 1$), and (5) stillborn baby ($N = 1$). A total of 10 nonchildbearing subjects dropped out during the study for the following reasons: (1) childbearing acquaintance dropped out ($N = 5$); (2) lost interest/too much work ($N = 3$); (3) moved away ($N = 2$).

Depression Outcome and Depression History Measures

Several self-report and interview-based measures were used in this study to capture the multidimensional nature of depression.

Self-Report Measures

The Beck Depression Inventory (Beck et al., 1961) was used as the primary measure of depressive symptomatology during pregnancy and the puerperium. The BDI has good psychometric properties, and it has been used frequently in general depression research (Rehm, 1988) and in research on postpartum depression (Cutrona, 1983; O'Hara et al., 1984). Approximately 7 of the 21 items on the BDI reflect somatic disturbances that frequently accompany pregnancy. Because somatic symptoms are greatly elevated relative to cognitive and affective symptoms in pregnant and postpartum women (O'Hara et al., 1984), for some analyses the BDI was divided into its cognitive–affective (items 1–14) and somatic (items 15–21) subscales.

The depression subscale of the SCL-90-R (Derogatis, 1983) was also used to measure depressive symptomatology because it has very few somatic items (2 of 13) and has been recommended for studies in which somatic distress might be high for reasons other than depression (e.g., with elderly or surgery patients) (Gallagher, Thompson, & Levy, 1980; Ghoneim et al., 1988). It is internally consistent and has high test-retest stability (Derogatis, 1983).

The Social Adjustment Scale-Self-Report, or SAS-SR (Weissman & Bothwell, 1976) is a 58-item questionnaire that assesses the subject's functioning in 6 role areas: work, friends, extended family, marital, parental, and family unit. One item referring to frequency of sexual intercourse was dropped from the marital subscale for comparisons involving childbearing and nonchildbearing subjects; however, 2 items reflecting enjoyment and problems with intercourse (e.g., pain) were retained. The measure is internally consistent and is stable over time (O'Hara et al., 1982). The measure has also been found to be significantly correlated with measures of depression in postpartum women (O'Hara et al., 1982).

The Visual Analogue Scales (VAS) were derived from the work of Cox and his colleagues (Cox, Connor, Henderson, McGuire, & Kendell, 1983; Kendell et al., 1981) and consist of 13 individual scales on which subjects rate a variety of mood states, such as depression, tearfulness, irritability, lability, elation, and relaxation (see Table 3.2). Each of the 8 negative mood and 5 positive mood scales (some of which were specially developed for this study) consists of a descriptive statement (e.g., "I have been feeling miserable and depressed") followed by a 100 mm line anchored on one end by "Not at all" and on the other end by "Worse (better) than I have *ever* felt before." The time frame for rating items was the past 24 hours. The 2 composite scores reported in the present study, VAS negative mood and VAS positive mood, represented the mean of the 8 negative and 5 positive scales, respectively. Visual analogue scales have been used in previous studies of the postpartum blues and depression (Cox et al., 1983; Kendell et al., 1981), and they have shown the expected pattern of increasing dysphoric mood in the first postpartum week. Moreover, they have also distinguished between childbearing women and female surgical patients (Levy, 1987).

The Premenstrual Assessment Form, or PAF (Halbreich, Endicott, & Nee, 1982), was used as an index of premenstrual depression in the current study. There are approximately 12 premenstrual syndromes assessed by the PAF (Endicott, Halbreich, Schacht, & Nee, 1981); however, our interest was in only 1 category, premenstrual major depression syndrome, because its criteria were derived from RDC major depression criteria. The items making up the premenstrual major depression syndrome show adequate internal consistency (Endicott et al., 1981).

Interview-Based Measures

The Research Diagnostic Criteria (Spitzer et al., 1978) were used to establish diagnoses of depression during the second trimester of pregnancy and the first 9 weeks postpartum. The RDC were also used to establish lifetime diagnoses of depression, hypomania, generalized anxiety disorder, and alcoholism. DSM-III (APA, 1980) criteria were used to establish diagnoses of dysthymia and cyclothymia.

Symptoms of current depression were assessed during a semistructured interview (O'Hara et al., 1984) adapted from the Schedule of Affective Disorders and Schizophrenia (Endicott & Spitzer, 1978). For diagnoses of current major depression, 8 categories of symptoms were rated by the clinician interviewer on 6-point scales (derived from the SADS) during the prepartum and postpartum interviews. A rating of at least 3 on a

6-point scale was necessary for a symptom to be counted as present. The 8 categories were comprised of 4 somatic symptoms (i.e., appetite disturbance, sleep disturbance, fatigue, motor disturbance) and 4 cognitive–affective symptoms (i.e., loss of interest, guilt, impaired concentration, suicidal ideation). Increased and decreased appetite and sleep were rated separately, as were agitated and retarded motor disturbance. This approach resulted in a total of 11 individual symptoms (7 somatic and 4 cognitive–affective) that were rated.

For all symptoms 2 ratings were made: (1) the absolute level of symptom severity; and (2) the level of symptom severity, adjusted for expected changes in pregnancy and the puerperium. Following the general SADS/RDC rule, a symptom that could be accounted for by another condition (e.g., physical illness) was not counted as evidence for a particular syndrome. A number of questions were asked to determine if symptoms were primarily attributable to childbearing. Did mood and symptom covary? Was the symptom present long before the mood disturbance? If sleep disturbance was evident, we asked whether the subject was getting up frequently to urinate or whether she was disturbed by the baby's kicking. During the postpartum period, if sleep disturbance was associated with frequent nighttime feedings, it was usually discounted. Overall, if there was no evidence that mood disturbance was responsible for the symptom, the adjusted rating was usually downgraded to a 1 or 2. For example, a woman who did not report much dysphoria yet reported significant fatigue would have received a high absolute rating for fatigue but a lower adjusted rating. With respect to cognitive symptoms, for example, a woman who reported little interest in usually pleasurable activities but who also reported a great deal of fatigue in the absence of dysphoria would receive a high absolute rating for loss of pleasure but a lower adjusted rating. The adjusted ratings were used as the basis for diagnostic decisions.

For lifetime diagnoses an adaptation of the SADS-L (Endicott & Spitzer, 1978) was used. The diagnoses of depression and other disorders in first-degree relatives and the subject's spouse were based on the Family History Research Diagnostic Criteria, or FH-RDC (Andreasen, Endicott, Spitzer, & Winokur, 1977). These criteria were assessed in the context of a semistructured interview. The FH-RDC has been found to be a reliable and valid method for assessing psychopathology in relatives (Andreasen et al., 1977).

Two indices of the postpartum blues were obtained. The first was based on the work of Pitt (1973). The blues were defined by the presence of both significant tearfulness and low mood lasting at least part of a day in the first 10 days postpartum (Pitt Criteria). A second set of criteria was derived from the work of Handley (Handley et al., 1980). The severity of 7 symptoms, including dysphoric mood, mood lability, crying, anxiety,

TABLE 3.2. Visual analogue scales.

On this sheet there are 13 scales describing different feelings you have experienced over the past 24 hours. Think back over the past day and place a mark on each line corresponding to the degree to which you felt the way described for each item.

Example

I have been excited.

✓ ____

Not at all | Better than I have *ever* felt before

If you did not feel very excited over the past 24 hours, you would have put your check mark nearer to the end that said "Not at all" (as shown above). If you had been very excited over the past day, you would have placed your check mark nearer to the end labeled "Better than I have *ever* felt before."

1. I have been feeling happy and self-confident.

____

Not at all | Better than I have *ever* felt before

2. I have been feeling miserable and depressed.

____

Not at all | Worse than I have *ever* felt before

3. I have been in tears.

____

Not at all | All of the time

4. I have been very worried and anxious.

____

Not at all | Worse than I have *ever* been before

5. I have been very irritable and quick tempered.

____

Not at all | Worse than I have *ever* been before

6. My spirits have been going up and down like a yo-yo.

____

Not at all | More so than I can *ever* remember

7. I have had experiences of suddenly feeling very frightened or panicky.

____

Not at all | Worse than I have *ever* been before

8. I have been tired and without energy.

____

TABLE 3.2. *Continued*

	Not at all	Worse than I have *ever* felt before
9. I have felt very useless.		
	Not at all	Worse than I have *ever* felt before
10. I have been relaxed and at ease.		
	Not at all	Better than I have *ever* felt before
11. I have been elated and on top of the world.		
	Not at all	Better than I have *ever* been before
12. I have been energetic and alert.		
	Not at all	Better than I have *ever* been before
13. I have felt confident and assured.		
	Not at all	Better than I have *ever* been before

insomnia, loss of appetite, and irritability, was assessed during the first 10 days postpartum. The interview to assess these symptoms was modeled after the SADS assessment of depression (see Table 3.3). Subjects met Handley criteria for the blues if they were rated as having 4 of 7 symptoms of at least mild severity (3 on a 6-point scale).

Interrater Reliability of RDC Diagnoses

In a previous study (O'Hara et al., 1984), we obtained very high reliability for diagnoses of current major and minor depression (kappa = 1.00) and past major depression (kappa = .95). The reliabilities of the absolute and adjusted cognitive and somatic ratings, also evaluated in an earlier study (O'Hara et al., 1984), were high as well (intraclass correlation range = .87 − .91). For the current study, the reliability for current major and minor depression based on 49 interviews was also high (kappa = .93). The reliability of past major depression was satisfactory as well (kappa = .92). Based on ratings of 46 relatives, there was perfect agreement with respect to depression in first-degree relatives.

TABLE 3.3. Interview to assess postpartum blues according to Handley criteria.

NOW THINK ABOUT THE DAY OR SEVERAL DAYS DURING THE FIRST WEEK TO 10 DAYS AFTER DELIVERY WHEN YOU FELT THE WORST. I WOULD LIKE TO ASK YOU SOME SPECIFIC QUESTIONS ABOUT THAT TIME.

1. Dysphoric Mood

HOW WOULD YOU DESCRIBE YOUR MOOD? DID YOU FEEL DEPRESSED (SAD, BLUE, MOODY, DOWN, EMPTY, AS IF YOU DIDN'T CARE)?

1—no evidence of blues
2—slight
3—mild—was depressed at least part of day
4—moderate
5—severe
6—extreme—very depressed for several days

2. Mood Lability

DID YOU HAVE THE EXPERIENCE DURING THAT TIME OF HAVING YOUR MOODS CHANGE EASILY? DESCRIBE THAT TO ME.

1—no mood change
2—slight
3—mild mood change—definitely noticeable to woman
4—moderate
5—severe
6—extreme mood change—changes dramatic and frequent

3. Crying

DID YOU HAVE CRYING EPISODES DURING THIS TIME? HOW FREQUENT WERE THEY?

1—none
2—just one or two mild ones
3—at least one intense crying episode
4—frequent crying, one day or so
5—frequent crying over several days
6—persistent crying over several days

4. Anxiety

DID YOU FEEL NERVOUS, ON EDGE, ANXIOUS, OR UPTIGHT DURING THIS TIME?

1—no anxiety
2—slight
3—mild—woman definitely aware of feeling anxious
4—moderate
5—severe
6—extreme—anxiety totally debilitating

5. Insomnia

TELL ME ABOUT ANY DIFFICULTY IN SLEEPING DURING THAT TIME NOT ASSOCIATED WITH FEEDING YOUR BABY.

1—none
2—slight—some small difficulty (less than a 1 hour delay)
3—mild—more than an hour delay (over at least 3 days)
4—moderate—more than $1\frac{1}{2}$ hour delay
5—severe
6—extreme—practically not sleeping

6. Loss of Appetite

HOW WAS YOUR APPETITE DURING THIS TIME?

1—normal
2—slight decrease

TABLE 3.3. *Continued*

3—mild decrease—definitely noticeable
4—moderate decrease
5—severe decrease
6—extreme decrease—practically no appetite at all

7. Irritability

DID YOU FEEL ESPECIALLY IRRITATED OR ANGRY WITH PEOPLE DURING THIS TIME?

1—not at all
2—slight
3—mild—definitely aware of irritability
4—moderate
5—severe
6—extreme—irritable and angry all of the time

Note: Questions in capital letters are the specific questions asked by the interviewer.

SOCIAL AND COGNITIVE VULNERABILITY MEASURES

The Dyadic Adjustment Scale (Spanier, 1976) is a 32-item instrument that was used to assess subjects' relationships with their partners. It has 4 reliable subscales: dyadic consensus, satisfaction, cohesion, and affectional expression. Items are rated on 2- to 7-point scales (e.g., "Do you and your mate engage in outside interests together?" ["all of them" to "none of them"—5-point scale]). In the initial validation study, the mean total score for married couples was 114.8 (SD = 17.8). The measure shows good internal consistency (alpha = .91) and has been shown to distinguish during pregnancy between women who do and do not go on to develop postpartum depression (O'Hara, 1986). Moreover, it has been commonly used in marital therapy outcome studies (Margolin, Michelli, & Jacobson, 1988).

The Self-Control Questionnaire (O'Hara et al., 1982; Rehm et al., 1981) is a 41-item instrument designed to assess subjects' attitudes and beliefs about their own self-control behaviors. Subjects respond on a 7-point Likert-type scale, indicating their degree of agreement with each item (e.g., "I am aware of my accomplishments each day"). The SCQ is internally consistent (alpha = .86) and was found to be stable over a 5-week period, $r = .82$ (O'Hara, 1978). The SCQ has correlated significantly with both prepartum and postpartum depression levels (O'Hara et al., 1982; O'Hara et al., 1984).

LIFE-STRESS MEASURES

The Pilkonis Life Events Schedule (Pilkonis et al., 1985) was used to index stressful life events during pregnancy and the puerperium. In earlier work the number of life events occurring during pregnancy and the first 9 weeks postpartum has been found to be associated with diagnosis of postpartum depression (O'Hara et al., 1984). In the current study, 92 of the 98 events from the PLES were used. Subjects were also asked about any events that were not listed. The number of negative events occurring between the beginning of pregnancy and the postpartum interview was used as the life events measure.

The Childcare Stress Inventory (Cutrona, 1983) was developed to index stressful postpartum events specifically related to childcare (e.g., baby has health problems) (see Appendix A). The number of childcare-related stressors indexed by the CSI has been found to be related to level of postpartum depressive symptomatology (Cutrona, 1983; O'Hara et al., 1984) and diagnosis of postpartum depression (O'Hara et al., 1984).

The Peripartum Events Scale (O'Hara et al., 1986) was completed for subjects based on their hospital charts after delivery (see Appendix B). The PES was developed to quantify stressful events related to pregnancy, labor, and delivery. Peripartum events are classified within the following subscales: medical risk factors, obstetric risk factors, indication for admission to labor and delivery, progress in labor, method of delivery, duration of labor, fetal monitoring, delivery complications, and infant outcome. The total score is the total number of events from these subscales. The measure has been found to be a reliable and valid measure of peripartum stress (O'Hara et al., 1986).

Social Support

The Social Support Interview (Mueller, 1980; O'Hara, 1986) is a 10-item scale that was designed to assess prepartum and postpartum social support provided by and given to a subject's spouse, closest confidant, and closest parent. Each question was asked separately for each of these 3 individuals (see Appendix C). Subjects were asked questions regarding the giving and receiving of instrumental support (e.g., helping with household tasks, childcare) and emotional support as well a mutual sharing of problems. Subjects were also asked about the extent to which they felt free to talk about anything they wished with each of these 3 individuals, how often each was available when needed, the extent to which each made the subjects' lives easier or more difficult, and the extent to which the subjects anticipated being able to rely on their spouses, confidants, and parents for childcare help after delivery. The same questions were asked during the postpartum interview.

The 3 subscales of the SSI (confidant, parent, and spouse) each show adequate internal consistency for (alpha = .77 to .85). Test-retest stability was assessed separately for childbearing and nonchildbearing subjects between the second-trimester interview and the 9-weeks postpartum interview (approximately 7 months). For the childbearing subjects, the stability indices were: confidant, $r = .436$; parent, $r = .672$; and spouse, $r = .440$. For the nonchildbearing subjects, the stability indices were:

confidant, $r = .514$; parent, $r = .713$; and spouse, $r = .647$. Evidence for the validity of the measure comes from two earlier studies that found that the SSI items distinguished between postpartum depressed and non-depressed women (O'Hara, 1986; O'Hara et al., 1983).

The Postpartum Social Support Questionnaire PSSQ (Hopkins, 1984) was designed to assess support provided to a new mother by several groups of individuals: spouse (18 items), parents (11 items), parents-in-law (10 items), other relatives (8 items), and friends (13 items). The measure asks subjects to rate the extent to which social network members provide a variety of types of support, including help with childcare and home maintenance, being available for confiding, and providing verbal expressions of support. Each of the 63 items is rated twice on 7-point scales ranging from 1 (almost never) to 7 (very often). Subjects first rate how often an individual (e.g., a spouse) provides a particular type of support and then rate how often they would like it to occur. For each item a difference score is calculated, reflecting degree of dissatisfaction expressed by subjects regarding the rate at which supportive activities are engaged in by their spouses, relatives, and friends.

The measure has shown good internal consistency for all subscales (range, alpha = .65 to .94) and adequate test-retest reliability ($r = .70$ to .77 over 2 months) (Hopkins et al., 1987; O'Hara, 1986). With respect to validity, in an earlier study we found that several of its subscales differentiated postpartum-depressed and -nondepressed women (O'Hara, 1986).

Hormone Assays

Serum prolactin was measured in duplicate by radioimmunoassay (RIA), using reagents supplied by New England Nuclear Corporation (Boston, Massachusetts). At an average concentration of 51 µg/L, the intraassay coefficient of variation (CV) was 4%; the interassay CV was 7%. The sensitivity of the assay was <0.10 µg/L.

Serum progesterone and estradiol were measured by a double antibody technique using reagents supplied by Research Systems Laboratories (Carson, California). For progesterone at an average concentration of 2 nmol/L, the intraassay CV was 8%; the interassay CV was 10%. At an average concentration of 12 nmol/L, the intraassay CV was 5%; the interassay CV was 6%. At an average concentration of 70 nmol/L, the intraassay CV was 7%; the interassay CV was 9%. The sensitivity of the assay was <1 nmol/L. For estradiol at an average concentration of 210 pmol/L, the intraassay CV was 7%; the interassay CV was 11%. At an average concentration of 720 pmol/L, the intraassay CV was 5%; the interassay CV was 10%. At an average concentration of 2930 pmol/L, the intraassay CV was 6%; the interassay CV was 11%. The sensitivity of the assay was less than 40 pmol/L.

Free and total estriol levels were measured using Coat-A-Count kits obtained from Diagnostic Products Corporation (Los Angeles, California). For free estriol at an average concentration of 5 nmol/L, the intraassay CV was 5%; the interassay CV was 6%. At an average concentration of 70 nmol/L, the intraassay CV was 5%; the interassay CV was 6%. The sensitivity of the assay was <1 nmol/L. For total estriol at an average concentration of 62 nmol/L, the intraassay CV was 4%; the interassay CV was 6%. At an average concentration of 695 nmol/L, the intraassay CV was 6%; the interassay CV was 8%. The sensitivity of the assay was <3 nmol/L.

Cortisol and urinary free cortisol were measured by RIA, using an antiserum obtained from American Biosystems (Marine, Minnesota) and I^{125} cortisol obtained from Research Systems Laboratories (Carson, California). For cortisol at an average concentration of 80 nmol/L, the intraassay CV was 8%; the interassay CV was 12%. At an average concentration of 610 nmol/L, the intraassay CV was 6%; the interassay CV was 7%. The sensitivity of the assay was approximately 30 nmol/L. For urinary free cortisol at an average concentration of 125 nmol/d, the intraassay CV was 5%; and at 165 nmol/d, the intraassay CV was 4%. The sensitivity of the assay was approximately 1 µg/liter, dependent on urine volume.

Procedure

Pregnant subjects and controls were recruited in the manner described earlier. Acquaintance controls were then yoked to their pregnant friends, such that each time a childbearing subject completed an assessment, her acquaintance control completed the same assessment at roughly the same time. The overall design of the study is portrayed graphically in Figure 3.1.

Subjects completed the BDI, SCL-90-R, Dyadic Adjustment Scale, SAS-SR, Self-Control Questionnaire, and Premenstrual Assessment Form and returned them by mail prior to their initial interview in the second trimester. Pregnant subjects and acquaintance controls completed the diagnostic interview in the Psychology Department, usually within 2 weeks of being recruited. Subjects also completed a BDI, SCL-90-R, and SAS-SR at 34 weeks gestation (third trimester). In addition, subjects completed the VAS at 34, 36, and 38 weeks gestation. These latter assessments were done in conjunction with blood and urine sampling. Prior to breakfast on these 3 occasions, 15 ml of blood was drawn. A 24-hour urine sample, ordinarily collected during the day prior to the blood draw, was also obtained.

Prior to breakfast and breast-feeding on days 1, 2, 3, 4, 6, and 8 postpartum, 15 ml of blood was drawn from each subject. A VAS was completed at the same time. On days 2 and 4 postpartum, 24-hour urines

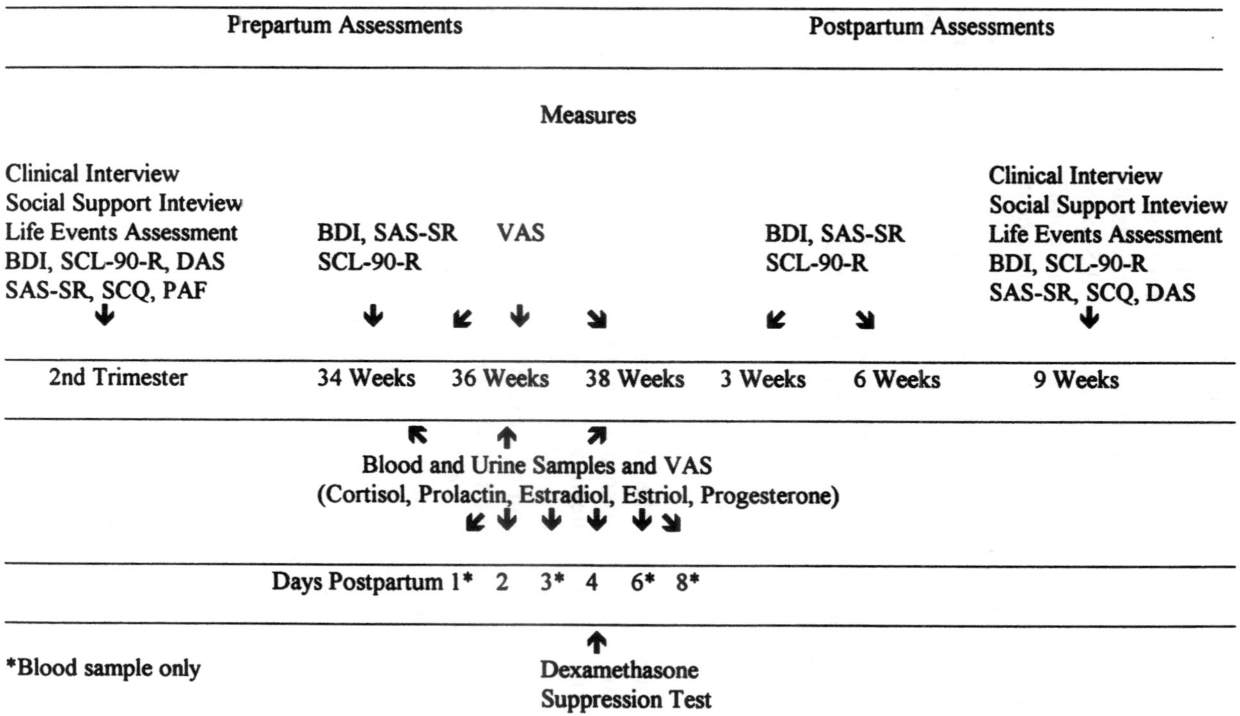

FIGURE 3.1. Design of prospective study of postpartum depression (BDI = Beck Depression Inventory; SCL-90-R = Symptom Checklist-90-R; DAS = Dyadic Adjustment Scale; SAS-SR = Social Adjustment Scale-self-report; SCQ = Self-Control Questionnaire; PAF = Premenstrual Assessment Form; VAS = Visual Analogue Scales; Interview = current and past psychopathology and family history of psychopathology).

were also obtained. Finally, on the evening of day 3 postpartum, a dexamethasone suppression test was begun. Subjects were given 1 mg of dexamethasone at 11:00 P.M. On day 4 postpartum, in addition to the morning blood draw, 7 ml of blood was obtained at 4:00 P.M.

The BDI, SCL-90-R, and SAS-SR were obtained again at 3, 6, and 9 weeks postpartum. The Childcare Stress Inventory was also completed at 6 weeks postpartum. At 9 weeks postpartum, subjects also completed the Dyadic Adjustment Scale, the Postpartum Social Support Questionnaire, and the Self-Control Questionnaire. As soon as possible following the return of the questionnaires completed at 9 weeks postpartum, subjects participated in a follow-up diagnostic interview focusing on the occurrence of depression since the initial interview in the second trimester and the occurrence of the postpartum blues. Social support from the woman's partner, confidant, and parent was also assessed along with life events that had occurred since the second-trimester interview.

Finally, at 6 months postpartum, the BDI, SCL-90-R, and SAS-SR again were obtained.

Summary

The major impetuses for the study were (1) the need to determine the extent to which the puerperium represented a high-risk period for depression; and (2) questions regarding the role of psychological, environmental, and biologic variables as risk factors for depression during pregnancy and for depression and the blues after delivery. A controlled prospective study was designed to answer these questions. The rest of this volume addresses the findings of our study. In chapters 4 and 5, changes over time in psychological functioning, social relationships, and life events of childbearing and nonchildbearing subjects are described. Chapters 6 through 8 report on the tests of our hypotheses regarding potential risk factors for depression during pregnancy and the blues and depression after delivery. Finally, the major findings of the study are summarized and the implications of these findings for our understanding of depression are discussed in chapter 9.

4
Psychopathology Across Pregnancy and the Puerperium

One of the major purposes of our study was to evaluate the adjustment of childbearing women across pregnancy and the puerperium as compared to the adjustment of a similar group of nonchildbearing women followed over a comparable period. In the next two chapters, the results of those comparisons will be described. In this chapter I will report on the personal and family history of psychopathology of childbearing and nonchildbearing subjects and the rates of diagnosed depression in the second and third trimesters of pregnancy and the first 9 weeks postpartum. The levels of depressive symptomatology and other types of psychiatric symptomatology in subjects across pregnancy and the puerperium will also be reported.

Clinical Depression After Delivery and During Pregnancy

In chapter 3 it was argued that in the early to mid-1980s the extent to which there was an increased risk for depression in the postpartum period was unclear. Rates of depression after delivery based on Research Diagnostic Criteria (Spitzer et al., 1978) or the DSM-III (APA, 1980) were found to range between about 8% and 14% (O'Hara & Zekoski, 1988). However, differences in diagnostic criteria, periods of time under consideration, and subject samples made it difficult to compare results from postpartum depression studies and epidemiological studies of depression (Myers et al., 1984). The inclusion of a carefully matched nonchildbearing control group allowed us to determine directly whether rates of depression were significantly increased during the postpartum period.

Although much of the research on psychiatric disturbance in childbearing women focuses on the postpartum period, and pregnancy appears to be a time of low risk for psychosis (Kendell et al., 1987), several studies have obtained relatively high rates of nonpsychotic depression during pregnancy as well (O'Hara & Zekoski, 1988). Pregnancy depression does not have the same distinction as postpartum depression;

however, data regarding its prevalence relative to rates of depression in nonchildbearing women are important.

Depressive and Other Psychological Symptomatology During Pregnancy and the Puerperium

Clinical depression represents a serious complication of pregnancy or the puerperium that can significantly disrupt a woman's functioning. However, clinical depression is defined on an all-or-nothing basis. Many women may experience a great deal of depressive symptomatology without meeting diagnostic criteria for depression. Numerous studies have included measures of depressive symptomatology for use during pregnancy and after delivery. The findings regarding the course of mood across pregnancy and the puerperium from these studies have been relatively consistent. Both self-report and interview-based measures of symptoms show a decrease in dysphoric mood from pregnancy to the puerperium (Cox et al., 1983; Elliott, Rugg, Watson, & Brough, 1983; O'Hara et al., 1984). The studies that have found an increase in symptom reports after delivery usually have conducted the first postnatal assessment early in the puerperium (Cox et al., 1983; Cutrona, 1983; Manly et al., 1982). These changes are often trivial in their extent and probably reflect symptoms of the blues.

One of the most thorough investigations of the course of mood changes across pregnancy and the puerperium was conducted by Elliott et al. (1983). They obtained self-ratings of mood (e.g., depression, tension, irritability, boredom, tiredness) on 7 occasions during pregnancy beginning about week 13, and on 11 occasions during the first year postpartum beginning at week 3. They included several self-report and interview measures; however, the findings from the self-report of symptoms are representative.

The only significant changes observed across pregnancy were increased worries about labor and decreased interest in and satisfaction with sex. Women also reported being more tired in the first trimester. After delivery, women reported significant decreases in most symptoms (e.g., depression, feeling fed-up, irritability, boredom, feeling unwell). Other mood measures were also congruent with these symptom ratings. During the postnatal year, once again, there was little change except for marked increases in sexual interest and satisfaction.

The findings from the Elliott et al. (1983) study suggest that women experience relatively stable mood across pregnancy and that mood improves after delivery and remains stable during the first postpartum year. Elliott et al. (1983) reported that pregnant women do not show symptom levels that are much above the median for normative samples of women who are not pregnant. For example, on the Eysenck Personality Questionnaire (Eysenck & Eysenck, 1975), the pregnant sample was not different from the normative sample on the Neuroticism Scale, and they were significantly lower than the normative group on the Psychoticism Scale. Nevertheless, there was significant variability among subjects in the pattern of mood change across pregnancy and the puerperium (Elliott et al., 1983). One limitation of the Elliott et al. study relevant to our work was the lack of a nonchildbearing control group. For example, it cannot be assumed that a nonchildbearing group would show stable and low levels of depressive symptomatology over time. Nor can it be assumed that there are no effects on test scores of repeatedly taking the same measure over the course of pregnancy and the puerperium. Finally, the fact that symptoms improve after delivery is somewhat inconsistent with the assertion that symptoms are at normal levels during pregnancy. Because of these considerations, the use of a nonchildbearing control group was thought to be essential in order properly to interpret findings from the childbearing women. Our expectation was that childbearing women would have higher levels of depressive and other psychological symptoms during the third trimester and at the earliest postpartum assessments (3 to 6 weeks postpartum).

Results

Approach to Data Analysis

Because the nonchildbearing control subjects were acquaintances of and matched to individual childbearing subjects, the data obtained from the childbearing and nonchildbearing subjects were not independent (Hays, 1988). The McNemar test for related samples was used to compare percentages of childbearing and nonchildbearing subjects who met criteria for depression and the blues (Kenny, 1987). It is similar to the Pearson χ^2, except that it was used for two related samples rather than independent samples. Two-way analyses of variance (ANOVA's) were used to test hypotheses involving the psychopathology-relevant variables that were measured on several occasions across pregnancy and the puerperium. The factors, group (childbearing, nonchildbearing) and assessment occasion (usually second trimester, third trimester, 3 weeks postpartum, 6 weeks postpartum, and 9 weeks postpartum), were both within factors. Childbearing status (i.e., group) was a within factor because childbearing and nonchildbearing subjects were individually matched. Subject pairs who had any missing data for a particular measure were not included in these analyses. Also, because of amount of missing data from the 6-month postpartum follow-up assessment, the BDI and SCL-90-R from that assessment were not included in the ANOVA's. Significant main effects for group or the interaction term were followed up with paired *t*-tests comparing the childbearing and nonchildbearing subjects at each assessment occasion. The sample sizes for the paired *t*-tests were often larger than the sample sizes from the overall ANOVA's because all available subject pairs were included in the follow-up paired *t*-tests, even if they were not included in the overall ANOVA (because of some missing data).

Personal and Familial Psychopathology

Childbearing and acquaintance control subjects were compared on a number of indices of personal and familial psychopathology based on the interview assessments during the second trimester (see Table 4.1). There was no basis for predicting any differences between childbearing and nonchildbearing control subjects with respect to personal or familial psychopathology, and none was found. There were rather significant levels of lifetime psychopathology in these participants. Despite the fact that the average age of participants was only 27 years, between 36% and 40% of them met criteria for a past history of major depression (prior to pregnancy). The rates of dysthymia and cyclothymia were relatively low, and other disorders were relatively uncommon as well. For example, between 4% and 8% of subjects met criteria for lifetime history of generalized anxiety disorder, and between 7% and 8% of subjects met

TABLE 4.1. Personal and family history of psychopathology in childbearing and nonchildbearing control subjects.

	Group		
Variable	Childbearing (%)	Nonchildbearing (%)	McNemar's $\chi^2(1, N = 179)$
Past depression	36.8	40.2	1.10
Premenstrual major depression syndrome	28.6	22.3	2.22
Dysthymia	1.1	3.9	<1
Cyclothymia	1.6	3.9	<1
Hypomania	4.9	8.9	<1
Alcoholism	8.2	7.3	<1
Generalized anxiety	3.8	7.8%	<1
Depressed first-degree relative	37.9	38.0	<1
Depressed partner	12.1	11.2	<1

Note: None of the McNemar χ^2's were significant. All indices except premenstrual major depression syndrome were derived from the second-trimester interview. Premenstrual major depression syndrome was derived from the Premenstrual Assessment Form (Halbreich et al., 1982). From "Controlled prospective study of postpartum mood disorders: Comparison of childbearing and nonchildbearing women" by M.W. O'Hara, E.M. Zekoski, L.H. Philipps, & E.J. Wright, 1990, *Journal of Abnormal Psychology, 99,* 3–15. Copyright 1990 by the American Psychological Association. Reprinted by permission of the publisher.

criteria for lifetime history of alcoholism. None of the childbearing subjects, however, reported abusive drinking during pregnancy.

Thirty-eight percent of our subjects had first-degree relatives (i.e., parents or siblings) who met diagnostic criteria for unipolar or bipolar disorder. Many subjects had more than 1 depressed relative. Roughly 12% of participants had a spouse who had experienced at least 1 depressive episode.

These findings suggest that depression was very common in the life experiences of our subjects. The rates of depression reported for relatives and particularly for spouses probably represents a significant underestimate of the true rates because of limitations in subjects' ability to observe their family members and spouses over time (Andreasen et al., 1977).

Pre- and Postpartum Depression

The presence of major and minor depression was determined for the period of the second and third trimesters and the first 9 weeks postpartum. The diagnostic interview conducted in the second trimester focused on the previous month. The prevalence of depression in the childbearing subjects (7.7%) was about one-third higher than it was in the nonchildbearing subjects (5.6%); however, this difference was not significant, McNemar $\chi^2(N = 177) < 1$. In the context of the 9-week postpartum interview, subjects were asked about any depressive episodes that might have occurred between the first interview in the second trimester and delivery. These episodes were called third-trimester depressions and covered about a 4-month period, in contrast to the second-trimester interviews, which covered a 1-month period. Again, the rate of depression in the childbearing subjects (11%) in the third trimester was higher than the rate of depression in nonchildbearing subjects (8.7%), but that difference also was not significant, McNemar $\chi^2(N = 177) < 1$. With respect to postpartum depression, there was no significant difference between the childbearing (10.4%) and nonchildbearing control subjects (7.8%) over the first 9 weeks postpartum, McNemar $\chi^2(N = 177) < 1$. The rates of major and minor depression at each of the assessments are displayed in Table 4.2. Interestingly, the ratio of depressed childbearing subjects to depressed nonchildbearing subjects was similar at each assessment (range 1.26 to 1.37).

Depressive Symptomatology in Childbearing and Nonchildbearing Control Subjects

For the BDI there were main effects for group, $F(1, 154) = 15.48$, $p < .001$, and assessment occasion, Exact $F(4, 151) = 41.62$, $p < .001$; the

TABLE 4.2. Number and percentage of childbearing subjects with depression (during pregnancy and after delivery) and blues (postpartum), compared with nonchildbearing control subjects at same assessment.

	Assessment occasion			
	Second trimester		9 weeks postpartum	
Measure	Childbearing	Nonchildbearing	Childbearing	Nonchildbearing
Research Diagnostic Criteria diagnosis				
Major depression	9	7	8	6
Minor depression	5	3	11	8
Total	14	10	19	14
Total (%)	7.7	5.6	10.4	7.8
Blues				
Pitt criteria (%)			41.8	10.1
Handley criteria (%)			26.4	7.3

Note: From "Controlled prospective study of postpartum mood disorders: Comparison of childbearing and nonchildbearing women" by M.W. O'Hara, E.M. Zekoski, L.H. Philipps, & E.J. Wright, 1990, *Journal of Abnormal Psychology, 99*, 3–15. Copyright 1990 by the American Psychological Association. Reprinted by permission of the publisher.

interaction of these two factors was also significant, Exact $F(4, 151) = 10.64$, $p < .01$. Paired t-tests revealed that the childbearing subjects reported significantly more depressive symptomatology than nonchildbearing subjects at the second-trimester, $t(175) = 4.06$, $p < .001$, and third-trimester assessments, $t(172) = 5.44$, $p < .001$, and at 3 weeks postpartum, $t(170) = 4.68$, $p < .001$. By 6 weeks postpartum, there were no significant differences (see Figure 4.1). Figure 4.1 shows that the BDI total scores for the childbearing subjects were highest during pregnancy, peaking in the third trimester and declining steadily after delivery. The pattern for the nonchildbearing subjects was quite different. Their scores gradually declined from the first through the last assessment. The 6-month follow-up assessment revealed no difference between groups with respect to their total BDI scores.

Many of the symptoms found on depression inventories may in part reflect the normal experience of childbearing women. Disturbances in appetite, sleep, and energy are commonly seen in childbearing women. We found in an earlier study that the BDI, when completed by pregnant or recently delivered women, may be biased by the items reflecting normal somatic disturbance (O'Hara et al., 1984). To assess this possibility, the BDI was divided into items reflecting cognitive and affective symptoms (items 1–14) and items reflecting somatic symptoms (items 15–21). Cognitive and affective symptoms included items reflecting feelings of sadness, discouragement about the future, guilt, self-criticism, suicidal ideation, and loss of interest in usually pleasurable activities, among others. Somatic symptoms included items reflecting ability to work, energy level, sleep and appetite disturbance, weight loss, concern about health, and loss of interest in sex.

There were clear differences in the pattern of findings for the somatic and the cognitive and affective items. For the somatic items, there were main effects for group, $F(1, 154) = 53.03$, $p < .001$, and for assessment occasion, Exact $F(4, 151) = 52.28$, $p < .001$. The interaction was also significant, Exact $F(4, 151) = 33.81$, $p < .001$. Paired *t*-tests revealed that childbearing subjects had significantly higher somatic subscale scores than did the nonchildbearing subjects at the second-trimester, $t(176) = 7.86$, $p < .001$, and third-trimester assessments, $t(172) = 10.64$, $p < .001$, and at the 3-week, $t(170) = 7.42$, $p < .001$, and 6-week postpartum assessments, $t(162) = 2.65$, $p < .01$. The pattern of the BDI somatic scores was similar to that for the BDI total, but more exaggerated. The scores of childbearing subjects peaked in the third trimester and declined thereafter,

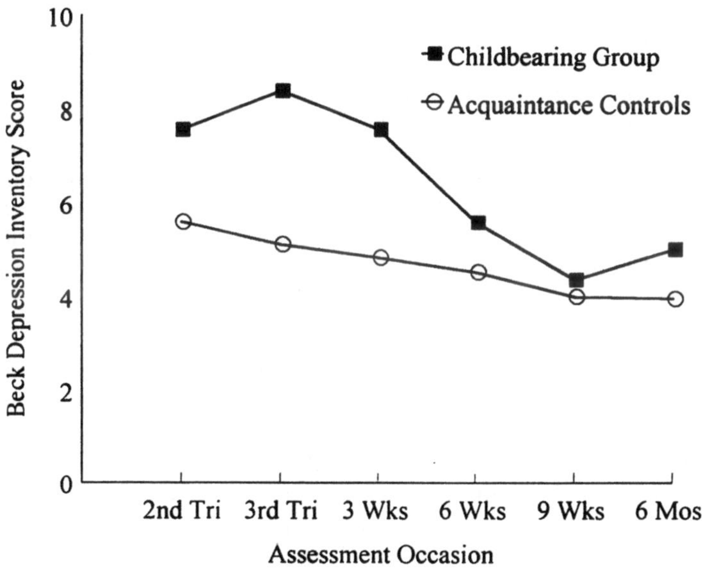

FIGURE 4.1. Beck Depression Inventory scores for childbearing and nonchildbearing subjects during pregnancy and after delivery. (2nd Tri = second trimester of pregnancy; 3rd Tri = third trimester; 3 Wks = 3 weeks postpartum; 6 Wks = 6 weeks postpartum; 9 Wks = 9 weeks postpartum; 6 Mos = 6 months postpartum.) From "Controlled prospective study of postpartum mood disorders: Comparison of childbearing and nonchildbearing women" by M.W. O'Hara, E.M. Zekoski, L.H. Philipps, & E.J. Wright, 1990, *Journal of Abnormal Psychology, 99*, 3–15. Copyright 1990 by the American Psychological Association. Reprinted by permission of the publisher.

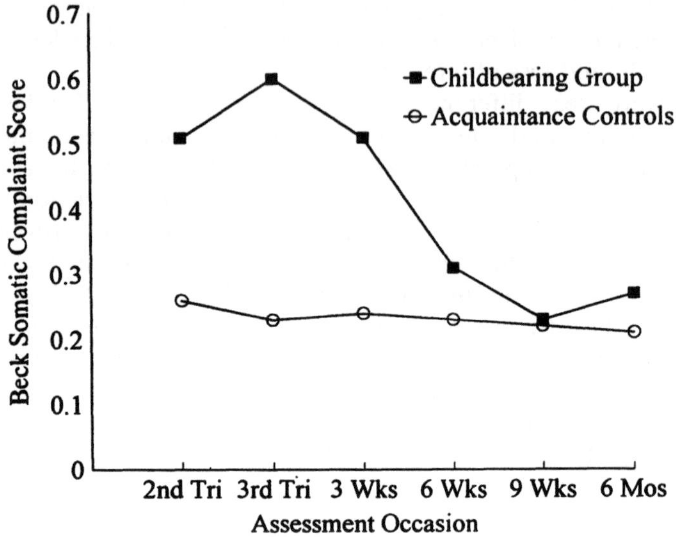

FIGURE 4.2. Beck Depression Inventory somatic complaint subscale scores for childbearing and nonchildbearing subjects during pregnancy and after delivery. (2nd Tri = second trimester of pregnancy; 3rd Tri = third trimester; 3 Wks = 3 weeks postpartum; 6 Wks = 6 weeks postpartum; 9 Wks = 9 weeks postpartum; 6 Mos = 6 months postpartum.) From "Controlled prospective study of postpartum mood disorders: Comparison of childbearing and nonchildbearing women" by M.W. O'Hara, E.M. Zekoski, L.H. Philipps, & E.J. Wright, 1990, *Journal of Abnormal Psychology, 99,* 3–15. Copyright 1990 by the American Psychological Association. Reprinted by permission of the publisher.

while the scores of the nonchildbearing subjects were low and stable throughout (see Figure 4.2). Also, no differences were evident at the 6-month follow-up.

The striking differences between childbearing and nonchildbearing subjects observed for the somatic items were not observed for the cognitive–affective items. There was a main effect for assessment occasion, Exact $F(1, 151) = 19.77$, $p < .001$; however, the group, $F(1, 154) = 2.44$, n.s., and the interaction effects were not significant, Exact $F(1, 151) = 1.65$, n.s. The overall pattern was similar to that for the BDI total but there was much less of a peak in the third trimester of pregnancy for the childbearing subjects (see Figure 4.3). There no differences at the 6-month follow-up as well.

We employed a second measure of depressive symptomatology: the depression subscale of the SCL-90-R (Derogatis, 1983). It was attractive in the current context because it has relatively few somatic items (2 of 13). There were main effects on this depression subscale for group, $F(1, 152) = 15.22$, $p < .001$, and for assessment occasion, Exact $F(4, 149) =$

31.91, $p < .001$. The interaction was also significant, Exact $F(4, 149) = 6.31$, $p < .001$. Paired t-tests revealed that the childbearing subjects had significantly higher depression scores than the nonchildbearing subjects at the second-trimester, $t(174) = 4.22$, $p < .001$, and third-trimester assessments, $t(172) = 4.77$, $p < .001$, and at the 3-week postpartum assessment, $t(170) = 4.78$, $p < .001$ (see Figure 4.4). There were no differences at the 6-month follow-up assessment.

The SCL-90-R taps a variety of dimensions of psychiatric symptomatology in addition to depression. No other subscale showed the same pattern as the depression subscale across assessment occasions. For example, even the somatization subscale revealed significant differences between childbearing and nonchildbearing subjects at the second- and third-trimester assessments only. Representative of the other subscales was the anxiety subscale. It contains items reflecting symptoms such as nervousness, trembling, feeling fearful, feeling tense, spells of terror, and the experience of thoughts or images of a frightening nature. Only at the third-trimester assessment did childbearing subjects report significantly more symptoms of anxiety than nonchildbearing subjects, $t(172) = 2.52$, $p < .05$ (see Figure 4.5).

Cognitive–affective and somatic symptoms of RDC-defined major depression were assessed during the prenatal and postnatal interviews.

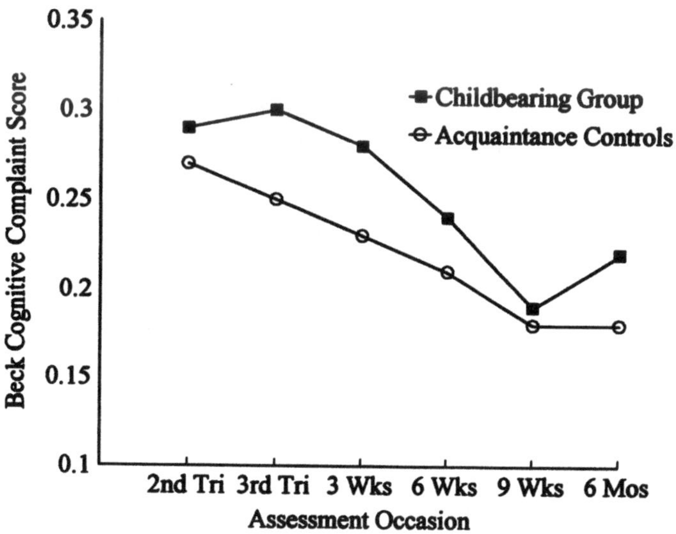

FIGURE 4.3. Beck Depression Inventory cognitive complaint subscale scores for childbearing and nonchildbearing subjects during pregnancy and after delivery. (2nd Tri = second trimester of pregnancy; 3rd Tri = third trimester; 3 Wks = 3 weeks postpartum; 6 Wks = 6 weeks postpartum; 9 Wks = 9 weeks postpartum; 6 Mos = 6 months postpartum.)

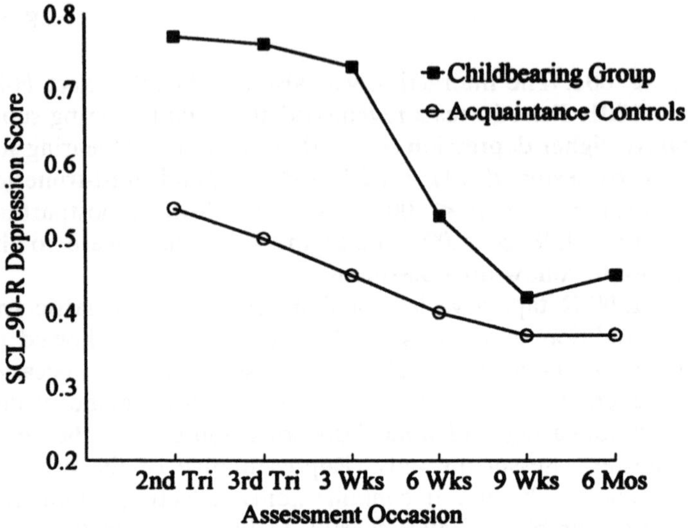

FIGURE 4.4. SCL-90-R depression scores for childbearing and nonchildbearing subjects during pregnancy and after delivery. (2nd Tri = second trimester of pregnancy; 3rd Tri = third trimester; 3 Wks = 3 weeks postpartum; 6 Wks = 6 weeks postpartum; 9 Wks = 9 weeks postpartum; 6 Mos = 6 months postpartum.) From "Controlled prospective study of postpartum mood disorders: Comparison of childbearing and nonchildbearing women" by M.W. O'Hara, E.M. Zekoski, L.H. Philipps, & E.J. Wright, 1990, *Journal of Abnormal Psychology, 99,* 3–15. Copyright 1990 by the American Psychological Association. Reprinted by permission of the publisher.

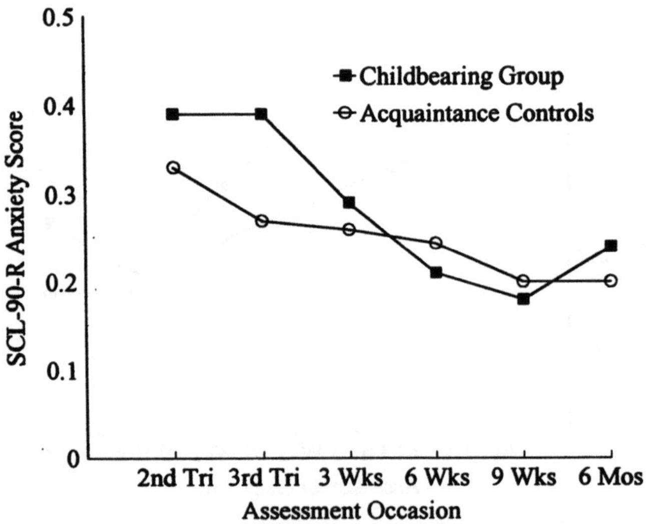

FIGURE 4.5. SCL-90-R anxiety scores for childbearing and nonchildbearing subjects during pregnancy and after delivery. (2nd Tri = second trimester of pregnancy; 3rd Tri = third trimester; 3 Wks = 3 weeks postpartum; 6 Wks = 6 weeks postpartum; 9 Wks = 9 weeks postpartum; 6 Mos = 6 months postpartum.)

TABLE 4.3. Cognitive and somatic symptoms of major depression defined by Research Diagnostic Criteria.

Cognitive–affective symptoms	Somatic symptoms
Loss of interest	Increased appetite
Guilt	Decreased appetite
Impaired concentration	Increased sleep
Suicidal ideation	Decreased sleep
	Fatigue
	Agitation
	Retardation

The specific symptoms included in each group are displayed in Table 4.3. In the last chapter, the process by which we took normal physical and psychological changes associated with pregnancy and the puerperium into account by adjusting the ratings of the somatic and cognitive–affective symptoms was described. These ratings were called the "adjusted" ratings; the parallel ratings for which no adjustments were made were called the "absolute" ratings.

For the absolute ratings (i.e., the unadjusted ratings) of cognitive symptoms, there was a main effect for group, $F(1, 176) = 11.98, p < .01$; however, the main effect for assessment occasion, $F(1, 176) = 3.85$, n.s., and the interaction, $F(1, 176) < 1$, were not significant. The paired t-tests revealed that childbearing subjects reported significantly higher absolute levels of cognitive symptoms than nonchildbearing subjects both before, $t(176) = 2.49, p < .05$, and after delivery, $t(176) = 3.13, p < .01$ (see Table 4.4). For the adjusted ratings of cognitive symptoms, there were significant main effects for group, $F(1, 176) = 5.30, p < .05$, and assessment occasion, $F(1, 176) = 7.19, p < .01$. The interaction effect was not significant, $F(1, 176) = 1.64$, n.s. Only at the postpartum interview, $t(176) = 2.42, p < .05$, did childbearing subjects report significantly higher adjusted levels of cognitive symptoms than nonchildbearing subjects (see Table 4.4).

For absolute levels of somatic symptoms, there were significant main effects for group, $F(1, 176) = 50.95, p < .001$, and for assessment occasion, $F(1, 176) = 12.51, p < .01$. The interaction effect was also significant, $F(1, 176) = 15.52, p < .001$. Paired t-tests revealed that childbearing subjects reported significantly higher absolute levels of somatic symptoms than nonchildbearing subjects at the prepartum, $t(176) = 7.81, p < .001$, and postpartum assessments, $t(176) = 3.55, p < .01$ (see Table 4.4). For the adjusted levels of somatic symptoms, there was a main effect for assessment occasion, $F(1, 176) = 10.53, p < .01$. The effects for group, $F(1, 176) < 1$, and the interaction, $F(1, 176) = 2.77$, n.s., were not significant (see Table 4.4). In summary, when the normal processes of pregnancy and the puerperium were taken into account,

TABLE 4.4. Means and standard deviations for interview-based ratings of absolute and adjusted ratings of cognitive and somatic symptoms.

	Cognitive–Affective		Somatic	
Group	Absolute	Adjusted	Absolute	Adjusted
		Second trimester		
Childbearing				
M	1.35	1.26	1.72	1.16
SD	.54	.49	.49	.39
Nonchildbearing				
M	1.23	1.21	1.32	1.19
SD	.40	.39	.46	.39
		9 weeks postpartum		
Childbearing				
M	1.43	1.37	1.51	1.28
SD	.61	.59	.50	.47
Nonchildbearing				
M	1.27	1.25	1.34	1.24
SD	.52	.51	.49	.44

Note: From "Controlled prospective study of postpartum mood disorders: Comparison of childbearing and nonchildbearing women" by M.W. O'Hara, E.M. Zekoski, L.H. Philipps, & E.J. Wright, 1990, *Journal of Abnormal Psychology, 99,* 3–15. Copyright 1990 by the American Psychological Association. Adapted by permission of the publisher.

the cognitive but not the somatic symptoms of RDC-defined major depression differentiated the childbearing and nonchildbearing subjects.

Mood During Late Pregnancy and Early Puerperium

In addition to the major measures of depression during pregnancy and the puerperium, we assessed the moods of subjects on 3 occasions late in pregnancy—weeks 34, 36, and 38 of gestation—and on 6 occasions after delivery—days 1, 2, 3, 4, 6, and 8 postpartum. We expected that the childbearing subjects would show significantly higher levels of dysphoric mood on days 3 through 8 postpartum, perhaps reflecting the postpartum blues. The Visual Analogue Scales that we used contained 2 subscales: the positive mood scale (5 items) and the negative mood scale (8 items) (see Table 3.2).

For the VAS positive mood scale, the main effect for group was not significant, $F(1, 118) < 1$; however, the main effect for assessment occasion was significant, Exact $F(8, 111) = 5.13$, $p < .001$. The interaction effect was also significant, Exact $F(8, 111) = 3.99$, $p < .001$. Paired *t*-tests revealed that the control subjects reported significantly more positive mood only at the 34-week gestation assessment, $t(164) = -3.32$, $p < .01$ (see Figure 4.6).

For the VAS negative mood scale, there was a main effect for group, $F(1, 122) = 8.54$, $p < .01$, and a main effect for assessment occasion,

Exact $F(8, 115) = 6.84$, $p < .001$. The interaction effect was also significant, Exact $F(8, 115) = 3.80$, $p < .01$. Paired *t*-tests revealed that childbearing subjects reported significantly higher levels of dysphoric mood at the 34-week, $t(166) = 3.12$, $p < .01$, 36-week, $t(161) = 3.71$, $p < .001$, and 38-week gestation assessments, $t(142) = 4.12$, $p < .001$; and at the day 4, $t(166) = 3.97$, $p < .001$, day 6, $t(166) = 4.06$, $p < .001$, and day 8 postpartum assessments, $t(164) = 4.31$, $p < .001$ (see Figure 4.7).

The negative mood symptoms were much more powerful than the positive mood symptoms in differentiating the childbearing and nonchildbearing women. Both the positive and the negative mood symptoms were rather stable across assessment occasions, as might be expected for the nonchildbearing subjects. The childbearing subjects showed increasingly negative mood during the third trimester. Their mood improved after delivery for 2 days but began to worsen until day 8 postpartum. The peak

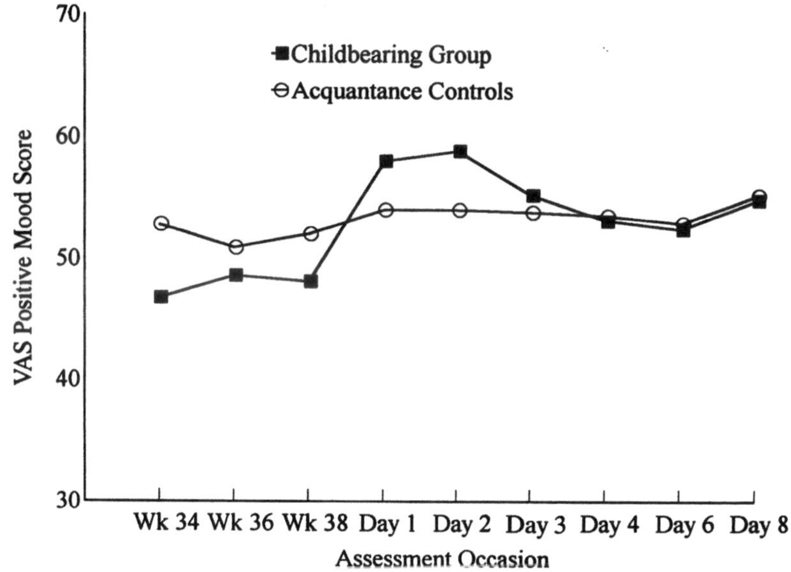

FIGURE 4.6. Visual Analogue Scales (VAS) positive mood scale scores for childbearing and nonchildbearing subjects during pregnancy and after delivery. (Wk 34 = 34th week of pregnancy; Wk 36 = 36th week of pregnancy; Wk 38 = 38th week of pregnancy; Day 1 = day 1 postpartum; Day 2 = day 2 postpartum; Day 3 = day 3 postpartum; Day 4 = day 4 postpartum; Day 6 = day 6 postpartum; Day 8 = day 8 postpartum. Range of VAS positive mood scale is 0–100; higher scores reflect more positive mood.) From "Controlled prospective study of postpartum mood disorders: Comparison of childbearing and nonchildbearing women" by M.W. O'Hara, E.M. Zekoski, L.H. Philipps, & E.J. Wright, 1990, *Journal of Abnormal Psychology, 99,* 3–15. Copyright 1990 by the American Psychological Association. Reprinted by permission of the publisher.

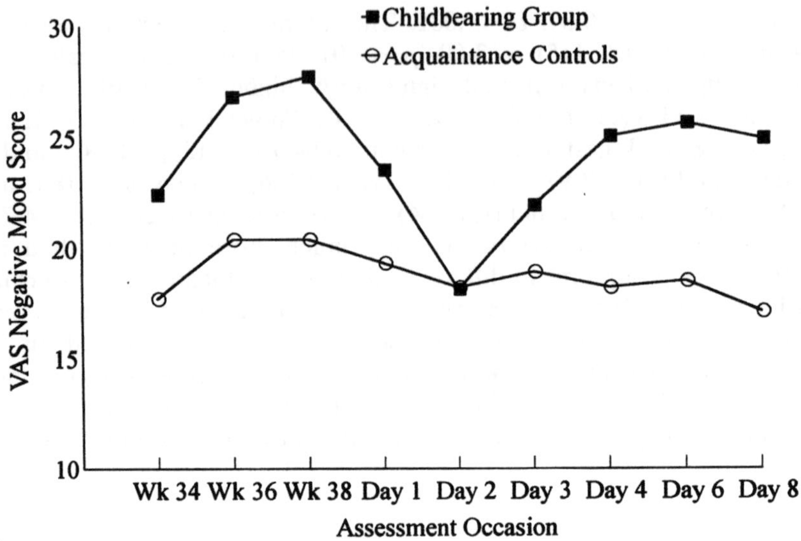

FIGURE 4.7. Visual Analogue Scales (VAS) negative mood scale scores for childbearing and nonchildbearing subjects during pregnancy and after delivery. (Wk 34 = 34th week of pregnancy; Wk 36 = 36th week of pregnancy; Wk 38 = 38th week of pregnancy; Day 1 = day 1 postpartum; Day 2 = day 2 postpartum; Day 3 = day 3 postpartum; Day 4 = day 4 postpartum; Day 6 = day 6 postpartum; Day 8 = day 8 postpartum. Range of VAS negative mood scale is 0–100; higher scores reflect more negative mood.) From "Controlled prospective study of postpartum mood disorders: Comparison of childbearing and nonchildbearing women" by M.W. O'Hara, E.M. Zekoski, L.H. Philipps, & E.J. Wright, 1990, *Journal of Abnormal Psychology, 99,* 3–15. Copyright 1990 by the American Psychological Association. Reprinted by permission of the publisher.

of postpartum dysphoric mood on days 4, 6, and 8 may reflect the postpartum blues, which are often seen to peak on day 5 postpartum.

Postpartum Blues

A significantly greater proportion of childbearing subjects than nonchildbearing subjects met Pitt criteria for the blues (i.e., presence of tearfulness and low mood), McNemar $\chi^2(1, N = 177) = 38.88, p < .001$. There was a similar outcome based on the Handley criteria for the blues (see Table 3.3), McNemar $\chi^2(1, N = 177) = 20.94, p < .001$ (see Table 4.2).

Childbearing subjects who met criteria for the blues were compared to childbearing subjects who did not meet criteria for the blues on the negative mood subscale of the VAS. It was expected that subjects who met criteria for the blues would have significantly higher levels of dysphoric mood after delivery, particularly on postpartum days 4, 6, and 8, than subjects who did not experience the blues. The first set of analyses concerned the Pitt criteria for the blues. For the VAS negative mood scale, there was a main effect for group, $F(1, 143) = 23.76$, $p < .001$, and a main effect for assessment occasion, Exact $F(8, 136) = 8.88$, $p < .001$. The interaction effect was also significant, Exact $F(8, 136) = 2.18$, $p < .05$ (see Figure 4.8). Independent *t*-tests (alpha level = .01) revealed that subjects meeting Pitt criteria for the blues reported significantly higher levels of dysphoric mood at the week 36 gestation assessment, $t(170) = 2.62$, $p = .01$, and at the day 2, $t(176) = 3.25$, $p = .001$, day 3, $t(177) = 4.29$, $p < .001$, day 4, $t(178) = 5.13$, $p < .001$, day 6, $t(177) = 4.09$, $p < .001$, and day 8 postpartum assessments, $t(176) = 4.57$, $p < .001$.

For blues defined by the Handley criteria, there was a main effect for group, $F(1, 143) = 17.34$, $p < .001$, and a main effect for assessment occasion, Exact $F(8, 136) = 7.17$, $p < .001$. The interaction effect was only a trend, Exact $F(8, 136) = 1.82$, $p < .10$ (see Figure 4.9). Independent *t*-tests (alpha level = .01) revealed that subjects meeting Handley criteria for the blues reported significantly higher levels of dysphoric mood at the 34-week gestation assessment, $t(174) = 2.67$, $p < .01$, and at the day 2, $t(176) = 3.12$, $p < .01$, day 3, $t(177) = 3.99$, $p < .001$, day 4,

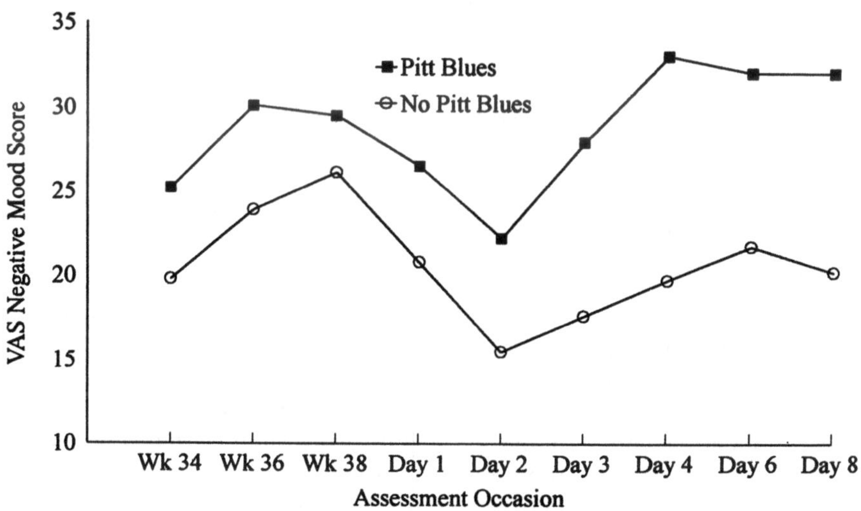

FIGURE 4.8. Visual Analogue Scales (VAS) negative mood scale scores for childbearing subjects meeting and not meeting the Pitt criteria for the "blues" during pregnancy and after delivery. (Wk 34 = 34th week of pregnancy; Wk 36 = 36th week of pregnancy; Wk 38 = 38th week of pregnancy; Day 1 = day 1 postpartum; Day 2 = day 2 postpartum; Day 3 = day 3 postpartum; Day 4 = day 4 postpartum; Day 6 = day 6 postpartum; Day 8 = day 8 postpartum. Range of VAS negative mood scale is 0–100; higher scores reflect more negative mood.)

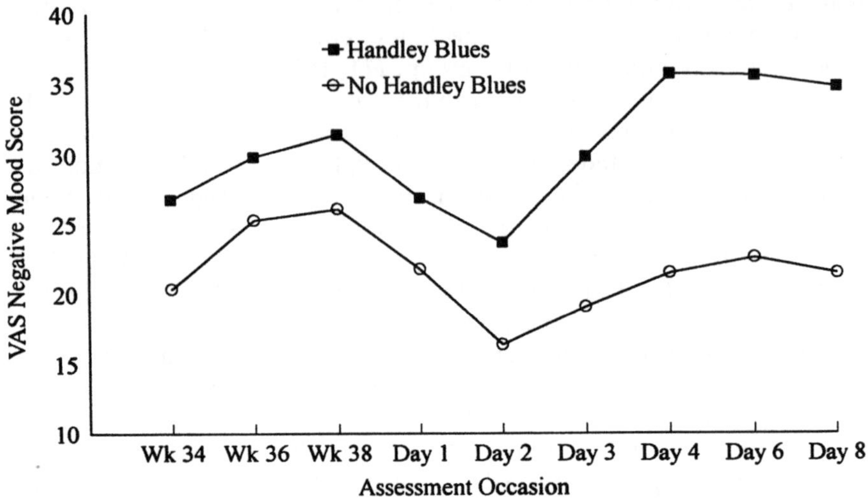

FIGURE 4.9. Visual Analogue Scales (VAS) negative mood scale scores for childbearing subjects meeting and not meeting the Handley criteria for the "blues" during pregnancy and after delivery. (Wk 34 = 34th week of pregnancy; Wk 36 = 36th week of pregnancy; Wk 38 = 38th week of pregnancy; Day 1 = day 1 postpartum; Day 2 = day 2 postpartum; Day 3 = day 3 postpartum; Day 4 = day 4 postpartum; Day 6 = day 6 postpartum; Day 8 = day 8 postpartum. Range of VAS negative mood scale is 0–100; higher scores reflect more negative mood.)

$t(178) = 4.80$, $p < .001$, day 6, $t(177) = 4.71$, $p < .001$, and day 8 postpartum assessments, $t(176) = 4.73$, $p < .001$.

Characteristics of "Postpartum"-Depressed Childbearing and Nonchildbearing Subjects

Differences in onset and duration of postpartum depression and symptom severity between depressed (major and minor, based on RDC) childbearing and nonchildbearing subjects were also explored. There appeared to be no differences with respect to when the depressions began. Three of the childbearing and 1 of the nonchildbearing subjects had depressions begin during pregnancy (see Table 4.5). One striking fact was that nine of the nonchildbearing subjects experienced depressions beginning within 8 days after the delivery of their childbearing acquaintance. In only 2 cases did matched childbearing and nonchildbearing subjects both experience a depression after delivery. There was no difference in the average length of an episode of depression between the childbearing (M = 45.9 days) and the nonchildbearing (M = 44.3 days) women, $t(32) < 1$.

Several indices of depressive symptomatology in postpartum-depressed childbearing and nonchildbearing subjects were examined in repeated measures ANOVA's. There were no significant main effects for group or interaction effects for the interview-based measures of cognitive or somatic symptoms. The depression subscale of the SCL-90-R showed a main effect for group, $F(1, 27) = 7.50, p < .05$. At the 3-week postpartum assessment, the depressed childbearing women had significantly higher SCL-90-R depression scores than the depressed nonchildbearing women, $t(30) = 3.56, p < .01$. For the BDI there were significant effects for group, $F(1, 25) = 5.09, p < .05$, assessment occasion, Exact $F(4, 22) = 3.67, p < .05$, and the interaction, Exact $F(4, 22) = 2.93, p < .05$. Depressed childbearing subjects had significantly higher levels of depression than depressed nonchildbearing women only at the 3-week postpartum assessment, $t(29) = 2.71, p < .011$ (see Figure 4.10).

For the somatic items on the BDI, there was only a main effect for group, $F(1, 25) = 3.66$, p< .01. The childbearing women had significantly higher somatic scores at the 3-week postpartum assessment, $t(29) = 3.24$,

TABLE 4.5. Onset and length of episodes of postpartum depression in childbearing subjects and nonchildbearing subjects.

Childbearing subjects			Nonchildbearing controls		
ID[a]	Onset[b]	Length[c]	ID	Onset	Length
003[a]	−95	165	006	25	10
012	2	21	009	1	14
015[a]	1	65	024	1	42
024	2	17	040	37	23
025	45	21	042	50	28
043	2	30	082[a]	35	21
045	11	7	086	5	10
070	1	69	091	8	21
082[a]	58	27	097	1	42
092	−30	120	103	5	64
123[a]	1	60	129	1	30
130	3	60	153	1	68
135	61	14	169	−153	240
144[a]	−30	95	188	3	31
155	16	8			
159	49	21			
166	44	21			
186	1	21			
189	3	31			

[a] These subjects all experienced an additional depression during the second trimester that remitted before delivery

Note: ID refers to subjects' identification numbers. A childbearing subject and her acquaintance control would share the same ID. Onset is in days relative to delivery or delivery of childbearing acquaintance. Length is in days.

Note: From "Controlled prospective study of postpartum mood disorders: Comparison of childbearing and nonchildbearing women" by M.W. O'Hara, E.M. Zekoski, L.H. Philipps, & E.J. Wright, 1990, *Journal of Abnormal Psychology, 99,* 3–15. Copyright 1990 by the American Psychological Association. Reprinted by permission of the publisher.

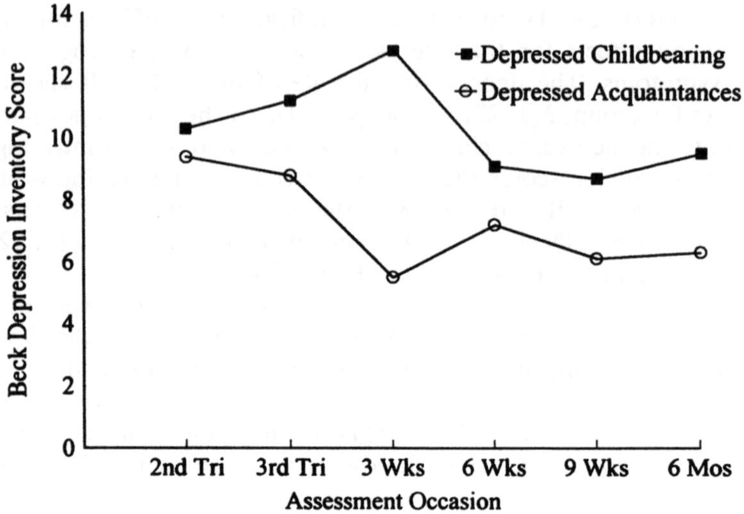

FIGURE 4.10. Beck Depression Inventory scores for childbearing and nonchildbearing depressed subjects during pregnancy and after delivery. (2nd Tri = second trimester of pregnancy; 3rd Tri = third trimester; 3 Wks = 3 weeks postpartum; 6 Wks = 6 weeks postpartum; 9 Wks = 9 weeks postpartum; 6 Mos = 6 months postpartum.) From "Controlled prospective study of postpartum mood disorders: Comparison of childbearing and nonchildbearing women" by M.W. O'Hara, E.M. Zekoski, L.H. Philipps, & E.J. Wright, 1990, *Journal of Abnormal Psychology, 99,* 3–15. Copyright 1990 by the American Psychological Association. Reprinted by permission of the publisher.

$p < .01$. For the cognitive items, there was only a significant assessment occasion effect, Exact $F(4, 22) = 3.95$, $p < .05$.

Summary

Despite the fact that the rates of depression for childbearing women were 26% to 37% higher than for nonchildbearing women during pregnancy and after delivery, the differences were not significant. Also, there were no differences between the childbearing and nonchildbearing women with respect to the timing of onset or the duration of the "postpartum" depressions. Assessments of depressive symptomatology across the last 2 trimesters of pregnancy and the puerperium revealed that depressive symptomatology was most elevated in childbearing subjects relative to nonchildbearing subjects in the third trimester. This finding was particularly striking on the somatic subscale of the BDI. Improvement in depressive symptomatology in childbearing subjects after delivery relative to pregnancy was evident by 3 weeks postpartum; dramatic improvement was evident by 6 weeks postpartum. Differences in levels of depressive symptomatology between childbearing and nonchildbearing subjects had largely disappeared by 9 weeks postpartum.

Childbearing subjects did experience symptoms of the postpartum blues to a much greater extent than the nonchildbearing subjects. Based on the Pitt or the Handley criteria, the childbearing subjects were about 4 times more likely to have the blues than the nonchildbearing subjects. Examination of the results from the Visual Analogue Scales revealed that the negative mood scales were much more likely to differentiate the childbearing and nonchildbearing subjects than were the positive mood scales during late pregnancy and the early puerperium. Consistent with expectations about the timing of the postpartum blues, dysphoric mood after delivery peaked about day 6 postpartum in the childbearing subjects.

Implications

Postpartum Blues

The rate of postpartum blues defined by either the Pitt (1973) or the Handley et al. (1980) criteria were in the low part of the range found in earlier studies (39% to 84%) (O'Hara, 1987). Pitt (1973) reported a prevalence rate of 50% in England using the presence of low mood and tearfulness as the only criteria for the blues, as compared to our rate of 41.8%. Our modified version of the Handley criteria for the blues (see Table 3.3), which required 4 of 7 symptoms of at least mild severity during the first 10 days postpartum, were much more stringent than the Pitt criteria and resulted in a markedly lower prevalence rate for the blues (26.4%). Both sets of criteria differentiated the childbearing and nonchildbearing groups equally well. The ratio of childbearing to nonchildbearing subjects who met the Pitt criteria was 4.1:1, and the ratio for the Handley criteria was 3.6:1. Moreover, 87.5% of the childbearing subjects who met Handley criteria for the blues also met the Pitt criteria, suggesting that the Pitt and Handley criteria define different levels of severity for the blues. Finally, although later, in chapter 7, predictors of the blues using the Handley criteria and a VAS-based definition for the blues are discussed, our unpublished data suggest that the same factors tend to be associated with the blues whether defined by the Pitt or Handley criteria.

The VAS ratings were consistent with the findings from the interview assessments of the blues. The positive and the negative VAS scales were relatively stable across postpartum day 1 to day 8 for the nonchildbearing subjects. However, the childbearing subjects showed a pattern that was characterized by a peaking on the positive mood scale on day 2 postpartum and a peaking on the negative mood scale on day 6 postpartum (Kendell et al., 1981; O'Hara et al., 1990). Relative to pregnancy, the mood of childbearing women improves significantly after delivery; however, by about day 3 postpartum it begins a downward turn. This characteristic mood pattern may reflect the exhilaration of the childbirth and then its gradual diminution. Another possibility is that this pattern may reflect relief that the pregnancy is over and then the reintroduction of household and childcare responsibilities and their associated stressors (women are often discharged from the hospital about day 3 postpartum). Whether the blues reflect psychosocial or hormonal readjustment or both, the blues is unpleasant (if not long-lived) and women should be prepared for its occurrence.

Prepartum and Postpartum Depression

The findings of the current study confirmed what has been suggested by earlier studies: Depression does not show an increased prevalence after childbirth (Cooper et al., 1988). The results of this study also indicated that the rates of depression during the second and third trimesters of pregnancy for childbearing women were comparable to rates of depression in nonchildbearing women followed over a similar period of time. The rate of postpartum depression (10.4%) observed in this study is in line with earlier work in the same setting (8.2%, Cutrona, 1983; 12.1%, O'Hara et al., 1984), in Great Britain (13.0%, Cox et al., 1982; 13.8%, Cox et al., 1993; 14.9%, Kumar & Robson, 1984; 12.0%, Watson et al., 1984), and in Uganda (10.0%, Cox, 1983). Interestingly, Troutman and Cutrona (1990) obtained a much higher prevalence rate of postpartum depression (26%, though only 6% major depression) in adolescents (14 to 18 years old) as compared to similar sample of nonchildbearing adolescents (15%), though the difference was not significant. Other studies have reported higher rates of psychopathology in childbearing women; however, they have included anxiety and other disorders in addition to depression (18.5%, Nott, 1987). In summary, for adult women it would appear that, based on criteria such as the RDC, the prevalence of postpartum depression is between 10% and 15% and that this range is not significantly higher than what would be found for comparable nonchildbearing women (Cooper et al., 1988; O'Hara et al., 1990; Watson et al., 1984).

The characteristics of the depressed childbearing and depressed nonchildbearing women were similar. For example, there were no differences between depressed childbearing and nonchildbearing women with respect to date of onset or duration of "postpartum" depressions. In fact, it was observed that several of the nonchildbearing subjects who experienced a "postpartum" depression reported that their depression began within 8 days of their childbearing acquaintance's delivery. This coincidence in timing may be due to the fact that we used the delivery date of the acquaintance of the nonchildbearing women as a reference point in the postpartum diagnostic interview. Given that most depressions have a rather insidious onset, it is likely that many of the depressions reported by nonchildbearing subjects began somewhat earlier or later than they reported.

The only depression-related variable that differentiated depressed childbearing subjects from depressed nonchildbearing subjects was level of depressive symptomatology during the early puerperium. These differences were most pronounced at 3 weeks postpartum and probably reflect the consequences of being depressed, trying to recuperate from childbirth, and taking care of a new baby at the same time. The differences between depressed childbearing and nonchildbearing subjects with respect to depressive symptomatology were greatly diminished by 6 weeks postpartum.

Depressive Symptomatology During Pregnancy and After Delivery

The findings from the interview-based assessments of depression symptoms, the Visual Analogue Scales, the Beck Depression Inventory, and the SCL-90-R depression subscale all converged to suggest that late pregnancy and the early puerperium are a time of increased psychological distress for women. This assertion stands in contrast to one of the most salient findings of the study—that there were no differences in rates of depression in the childbearing and nonchildbearing groups.

These findings are similar to a recent study of women experiencing the chronic stress of caring for a handicapped child (Breslau & Davis, 1986). In this study there were no differences in rates of major depression between the women experiencing chronic stress and a large sample of randomly selected controls. However, the women experiencing the chronic stress reported significantly higher levels of depressive symptomatology, as measured by the CES-D. These findings and the findings of the current study together suggest that some events or stressful life circumstances are more predictive of increased psychological distress than of increased rates of major depression.

A major element of the distress experienced by childbearing women appeared to be directly related to many of the physical changes associated with pregnancy and childbirth. For example, the most dramatic differences between childbearing and nonchildbearing subjects were found on the somatic subscale of the BDI. Nevertheless, measures that had small loadings on physical complaints (e.g., SCL-90-R depression subscale) also showed significant differences between childbearing and nonchildbearing subjects.

Observation as Prevention or Therapy?

What might have been the effects of the intensive series of assessments that we carried out with study participants over the course of about 7 months? In addition to the personal interviews (second trimester and 9 weeks postpartum) in which subjects participated, staff contacted subjects to remind them to return questionnaires when they were due. The child-bearing subjects also had blood draws and urine collections during the third trimester and during the first week postpartum. There is some evidence that women exposed to frequent contact with research workers will have a lower rate of postpartum depression than women who have relatively little contact with research workers (Kumar & Robson, 1984). Staff did not attempt to provide therapy or even explicit support to subjects; however, they were rather sympathetic and attentive to subjects. Nevertheless, both the childbearing and nonchildbearing women received this attention. Although the overall rate of postpartum depression may have been lowered by our repeated contact with subjects, the effects should have been equally present in the nonchildbearing subjects, suggesting that the overall conclusions from this element of the study would not be altered.

5 Adjustment, Social Support, and Life Events Across Pregnancy and the Puerperium

Pregnancy and the puerperium were both associated with some increase in level of depressive symptomatology, particularly the third trimester of pregnancy and the first 3 weeks postpartum. These differences were reflected in a higher incidence of blues in the childbearing subjects in the first week after delivery but not in diagnosed depression during pregnancy or in the first 9 weeks after delivery. Although risk for depression in childbearing women was the major focus of our work, we were also interested in outcomes and processes that reflected social functioning and the women's interactions with their social environments. For example, does childbearing impact on a woman's relationship with her partner, family members, and friends?

Social Adjustment and Social Support

During pregnancy we might expect a woman to reexamine her relationships with respect to their impact on her ability to care for her baby. The increasing salience of the upcoming delivery as her pregnancy progresses should focus a woman's attention more and more on her relationships with her partner and other family members and perhaps less and less on her work and other social relationships. This process should be most potent during the early postpartum period, when the demands of childcare have become a reality. The course of the woman's relationship with her partner over pregnancy and the puerperium has been more frequently studied than other relationships. One relatively consistent finding is that the marital relationship tends to deteriorate after delivery relative to pregnancy (Belsky, Lang, & Rovine, 1985; Waldron & Routh, 1981). The cause of this deterioration in the marital relationship is not altogether clear. However, it may be that many women's expectations for their partners' involvement in childcare activities and household responsibilities are violated. These perspectives led us to predict that the marital relationship would be less satisfying to childbearing subjects than to nonchildbearing subjects during the postpartum period. We made no predictions regarding changes in social adjustment of childbearing women with respect to relationships with their other family members and friends or their ability to work.

Closely related to adjustment in social relationships is the social support that a woman receives from and provides to individuals such as her partner, parents, and close friends. Pregnancy and the early puerperium are times when it is traditional for members of a woman's social network, particularly family members, to provide extra help and support to ease her transition to motherhood (either again or for the first time). Women who receive support from their social networks and are able to provide support to others during pregnancy and the puerperium should be better adjusted in all of their major social relationships. Consistent with our predictions regarding the adjustment of women in their social relationships, we expected that childbearing women would report lower levels of social support from their partner relative to nonchildbearing women during the postpartum period. Again, we had no predictions regarding social support received from and given to parents and confidants.

Measures

Two measures of social adjustment and two measures of social support were obtained in this study. The Social Adjustment Scale-self-report was obtained on 6 occasions: the second and third trimesters, and 3 weeks, 6 weeks, 9 weeks, and 6 months postpartum. As we described in Chapter 3, the SAS-SR was designed to assess the social role functioning of women in the areas of work in and outside of the home, relationship with spouse, relationship with family members, relationship with children, and relationship with friends (Weissman & Bothwell, 1976). The Dyadic Adjustment Scale was the second measure of social functioning (Spanier, 1976). The DAS reflected the woman's relationship with her partner and was administered in the second trimester of pregnancy and 9 weeks postpartum. The repeated assessments with the SAS-SR and the DAS over pregnancy and the puerperium allowed us to document changes in social functioning associated with childbearing.

Social support was indexed with two measures: the Social Support Interview and the Postpartum Social Support Questionnaire. The SSI is a 13-item scale (see Appendix C) that asks a woman about support she provides to and receives from her partner, closest parent, and closest confidant and about the woman's general satisfaction with support (Mueller, 1980; O'Hara, 1986). The SSI was administered during the second trimester of pregnancy and at 9 weeks postpartum. The PSSQ was designed to assess social support provided to a new mother by her spouse, parents, in-laws, other relatives, and friends (Hopkins, 1984). It was administered only to childbearing subjects and only at the 9-week postpartum assessment.

Stressful Life Events

The occurrence of stressful life events during pregnancy or after delivery clearly would affect the adjustment of a childbearing woman. However, is there any reason to believe that childbearing women relative to nonchildbearing women would be at risk for increased levels of stressful life events? Although most stressful life events are independent of pregnancy and the puerperium, some events may be consequences of pregnancy or childbirth. For example, a couple may have housing that is inadequate for a new baby and be forced to move. The financial consequences of having a new baby may require the father to work extra hours or an additional part-time job (particularly if the woman stops working or takes an extended maternity leave). The time necessary to care for the new baby may reduce the time a woman has available to maintain her relationship with her partner and friends. Consequently, these relationships may become disrupted. A promising career or schooling may be interrupted by the birth of a child. Performance in many important activities (e.g., work, school) may be affected by the birth of a child. In summary, there are many stressful life events associated with pregnancy and childbirth that are social consequences rather than biological consequences (e.g., fatigue). Given these considerations, we expected that childbearing women would experience a higher level of negative events than nonchildbearing women, particularly during the postpartum period.

In addition to stressful events that are social consequences of pregnancy and childbirth, there are stressful events that are more tied to childbearing itself. These events include complications of pregnancy or delivery (e.g., eclampsia, difficult delivery) and problems with the newborn (e.g., difficulty establishing a feeding schedule). Of course, these are events that would not occur to nonchildbearing women; however, they are important to index because of their relevance to postpartum adjustment. Because we assessed these childbearing-specific life events in earlier studies, it was possible to compare the current sample of childbearing subjects to our subjects from earlier studies.

Measures

The Pilkonis Life Events Schedule was used to assess stressful life events experienced by childbearing and nonchildbearing subjects during pregnancy and through the first 9 weeks postpartum (Pilkonis et al., 1985). Events were assessed during the second-trimester and 9-week postpartum interviews. The two stressful life event measures specifically targeted to childbearing subjects were the Childcare Stress Inventory (Cutrona, 1983) and the Peripartum Events Scale (O'Hara et al., 1986) (see Appendices A and B). The CSI assesses the number and severity of childcare-related stressful events (e.g., baby has health problems) and it was obtained at 6 weeks postpartum. The PES was designed to quantify stressful events related to pregnancy, labor, and delivery. It was completed by an obstetrician who gathered the necessary information from each subject's medical record.

Results

Approach to Data Analysis

The same basic approach to data analysis that was described in Chapter 4 was employed in comparing the social adjustment, social support, and stressful life events of the childbearing and nonchildbearing subjects. Two-way ANOVA's were used to test hypotheses involving the adjustment, social support, and life event-relevant variables that were measured on several occasions across pregnancy and the puerperium. The factors—group (childbearing, nonchildbearing) and assessment occasion (second trimester, third trimester, 3 weeks postpartum, 6 weeks postpartum, and 9 weeks postpartum or second trimester and 9 weeks postpartum)—were both within factors. Subject pairs who had any missing data for a particular measure were not included in these analyses. Also, because of amount of missing data from the 6-month postpartum follow-up assessment, the SAS-SR's from that assessment were not included in the ANOVA's. Significant main effects for group or the interaction term were followed up with paired t-tests comparing the childbearing and nonchildbearing subjects at each assessment occasion. The sample sizes for the paired t-tests were often larger than the sample sizes from the overall ANOVA's, because all available subject pairs were included in the follow-up paired t-tests even if they were not included in the overall ANOVA (because of some missing data).

Social Adjustment in Childbearing and Nonchildbearing Subjects

The total score of the SAS-SR reflects the sum of all of the items that make up the various subscales, and it represents the most general index of social adjustment. For the total SAS-SR, there were main effects for group, $F(1, 157) = 8.90, p < .01$, and for assessment occasion, Exact $F(4, 154) = 26.92, p < .001$. The interaction effect was also significant, Exact $F(4, 154) = 3.56, p < .01$. Paired t-tests revealed that the childbearing subjects reported significantly poorer social adjustment than nonchildbearing subjects at the 3-week, $t(171) = 4.24$, $p < .001$, and 6-week postpartum assessments, $t(163) = 2.69$, $p < .01$ (see Figure 5.1). A separate analysis for the 6-month follow-up revealed no significant difference between childbearing and nonchildbearing subjects, $t(134) = 1.56$, n.s.

The three subscales reflecting adjustment in relationships with spouse, family, and friends were also analyzed. For the family relationship subscale of the SAS-SR, there was a significant effect for assessment occasion, $F(4, 151) = 13.33$, $p < .001$; however, neither the main effect for group nor the interaction effect was significant (see Figure 5.2). The occasion effect reflected a trend toward general improvement over time for both groups. For the relationship with friends subscale, there was a main effect for group, $F(1, 156) = 4.44$, $p < .05$, and a main effect for assessment occasion, $F(4, 153) = 6.10$, $p < .001$. The interaction effect was not significant, $F(4, 153) = 1.52$, n.s. For the relationships with friends subscale, the childbearing subjects reported a significantly poorer relationship with friends than the nonchildbearing subjects at the second-trimester

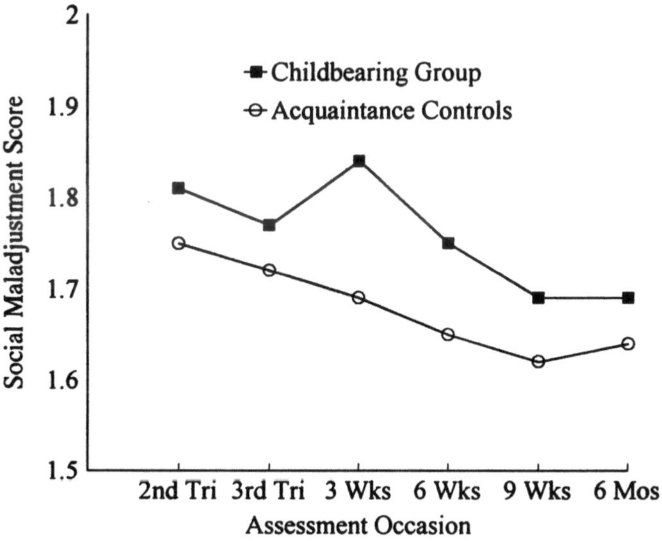

FIGURE 5.1. Total scores on Social Adjustment Scale-self-report (SAS-SR) for childbearing and nonchildbearing subjects during pregnancy and after delivery. (2nd Tri = second trimester of pregnancy; 3rd Tri = third trimester; 3 Wks = 3 weeks postpartum; 6 Wks = 6 weeks postpartum; 9 Wks = 9 weeks postpartum; 6 Mos = 6 months postpartum.) From "Controlled prospective study of postpartum mood disorders: Comparison of childbearing and nonchildbearing women" by M.W. O'Hara, E.M. Zekoski, L.H. Philipps, & E.J. Wright, 1990, *Journal of Abnormal Psychology, 99,* 3–15. Copyright 1990 by the American Psychological Association. Reprinted by permission of the publisher.

assessment, $t(176) = 3.20$, $p < .01$, and the 6-month follow-up assessment, $t(134) = 2.20$, $p < .05$ (see Figure 5.3).

For the marital relationship subscale of the SAS-SR, there were main effects for group, $F(1, 127) = 10.44$, $p < .01$, and for assessment occasion, Exact $F(4, 124) = 6.66$, $p < .001$. The interaction effect was not significant, Exact $F(4, 124) = 2.23$. The childbearing subjects reported significantly poorer marital adjustment than the nonchildbearing subjects at the third-trimester assessment, $t(144) = 3.00$, $p < .01$; at the 3-week, $t(145) = 3.53$, $p < .01$, 6-week, $t(136) = 2.92$, $p < .01$, and 9-week assessments, $t(145) = 3.03$, $p < .01$; and at the 6-month follow-up assessment, $t(113) = 2.33$, $p < .05$ (see Figure 5.4).

Marital adjustment was also indexed by the Dyadic Adjustment Scale, which subjects completed during the second trimester and at 9 weeks postpartum. For the DAS there was a significant interaction effect, $F(1, 153) = 8.35$, $p < .01$; however, neither the main effect for group, $F(1, 153) = 2.41$, nor the main effect for assessment occasion, $F(1, 153) = 1.24$, was significant. Paired t-tests revealed that childbearing subjects reported a significantly higher level of marital satisfaction than nonchildbearing subjects during pregnancy, $t(158) = 2.36$, $p < .05$, but not after delivery (see Table 5.1).

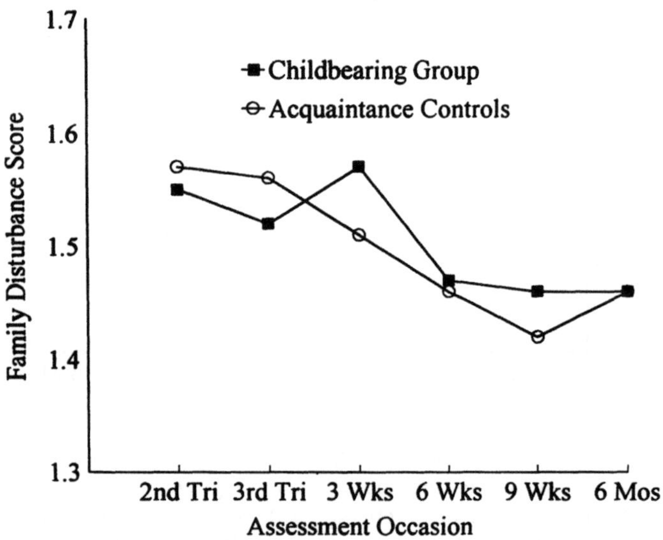

FIGURE 5.2. Scores on the relationships with family subscale of the Social Adjustment Scale-self-report (SAS-SR) for childbearing and nonchildbearing subjects during pregnancy and after delivery. (2nd Tri = second trimester of pregnancy; 3rd Tri = third trimester, 3 Wks = 3 weeks postpartum; 6 Wks = 6 weeks postpartum; 9 Wks = 9 weeks postpartum; 6 Mos = 6 months postpartum.)

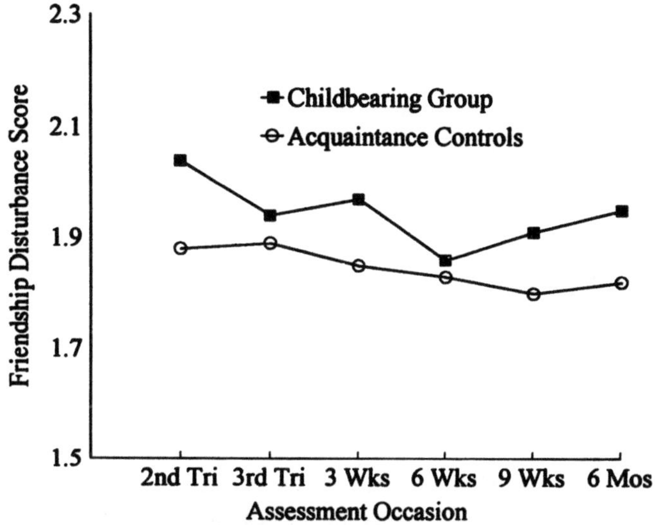

FIGURE 5.3. Scores on the relationships with friends subscale of the Social Adjustment Scale-self-report (SAS-SR) for childbearing and nonchildbearing subjects during pregnancy and after delivery. (2nd Tri = second trimester of pregnancy; 3rd Tri = third trimester, 3 Wks = 3 weeks postpartum; 6 Wks = 6 weeks postpartum; 9 Wks = 9 weeks postpartum; 6 Mos = 6 months postpartum.) From "Controlled prospective study of postpartum mood disorders: Comparison of childbearing and nonchildbearing women" by M.W. O'Hara, E.M. Zekoski, L.H. Philipps, & E.J. Wright, 1990, *Journal of Abnormal Psychology, 99,* 3–15. Copyright 1990 by the American Psychological Association. Reprinted by permission of the publisher.

Adjustment in work at home was also assessed by the SAS-SR. There was a significant effect for assessment occasion, Exact $F(4, 149) = 9.92$, $p < .001$; however, neither the main effect for group, $F(1, 152) < 1$, nor the interaction effect, $F(4, 149) = 2.13$, was significant (see Figure 5.5). The general trend for both groups was that adjustment tended to improve across the 6 assessment periods.

Social Support

At the second-trimester and 9-week-postpartum interviews, an assessment was made of the extent to which subjects received from and provided social support to (1) close confidants; (2) parents (usually mothers); and (3) partners. Among the childbearing women, 8.2% did not have anyone in whom they confided about themselves or their problems. The comparable rate for nonchildbearing subjects was 7.3%. With respect to the parent in whom subjects could most easily confide, mothers were most commonly selected (90.1% for childbearing and 79.9% for nonchild-

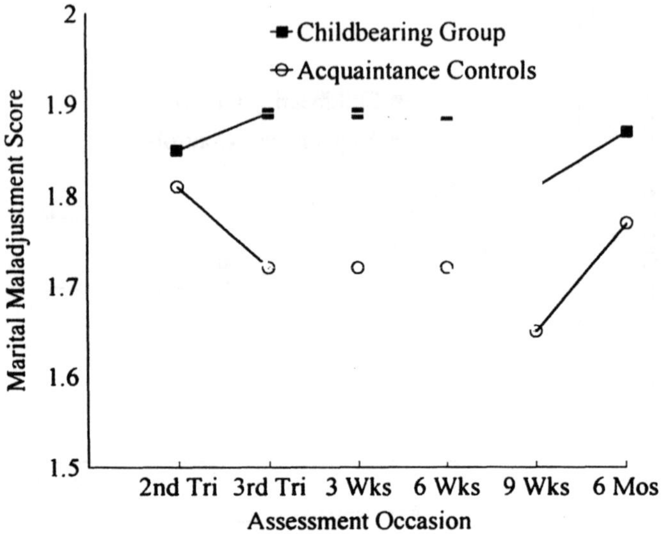

FIGURE 5.4. Scores on the martial adjustment subscale of the Social Adjustment Scale-self-report (SAS-SR) for childbearing and nonchildbearing subjects during pregnancy and after delivery. (2nd Tri = second trimester of pregnancy; 3rd Tri = third trimester; 3 Wks = 3 weeks postpartum; 6 Wks = 6 weeks postpartum; 9 Wks = 9 weeks postpartum; 6 Mos = 6 months postpartum.) From "Controlled prospective study of postpartum mood disorders: Comparison of childbearing and nonchildbearing women" by M.W. O'Hara, E.M. Zekoski, L.H. Philipps, & E.J. Wright, 1990, *Journal of Abnormal Psychology, 99,* 3–15. Copyright 1990 by the American Psychological Association. Reprinted by permission of the publisher.

bearing subjects). About 3% of both groups of subjects did not have parents available (usually because of death). With respect to partners, 7.1% of the childbearing women and 11.2% of the nonchildbearing women did not have partners available in whom they could confide.

TABLE 5.1. Means and standard deviations for the Dyadic Adjustment Scale during pregnancy and after delivery.

	Time of assessment	
Group	Second trimester	9 weeks postpartum
Childbearing		
M	114.00	112.70
SD	13.36	18.09
Nonchildbearing		
M	110.72	112.78
SD	16.55	15.71

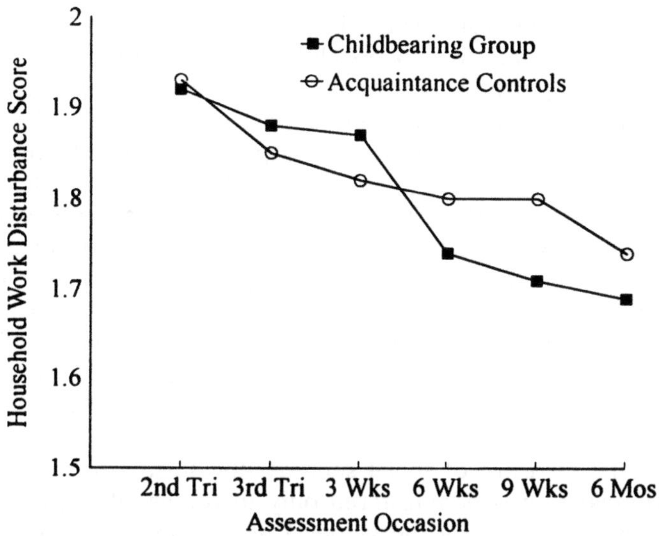

FIGURE 5.5. Scores on the household work subscale of the Social Adjustment Scale-self-report (SAS-SR) for childbearing and nonchildbearing subjects during pregnancy and after delivery. (2nd Tri = second trimester of pregnancy; 3rd Tri = third trimester; 3 Wks = 3 weeks postpartum; 6 Wks = 6 weeks postpartum; 9 Wks = 9 weeks postpartum; 6 Mos = 6 months postpartum.)

For support provided by subjects' confidants, there were main effects for group, $F(1, 137) = 6.69$, $p < .05$, and for assessment occasion, $F(1, 137) = 107.86$, $p < .001$; the interaction effect was not significant, $F(1, 137) = 1.12$ (see Table 5.2). Paired t-tests revealed that childbearing subjects reported less support from confidants at the time of the second-trimester interview, $t(146) = 2.08$, $p < .05$, and at 9 weeks postpartum, $t(147) = 2.49$, $p < .05$. Both the childbearing subjects, $t(153) = -8.47$, $p < .001$, and the nonchildbearing subjects, $t(158) = -7.51$, $p < .001$, reported significantly less social support from their confidants at 9 weeks postpartum relative to the second trimester of pregnancy.

For support provided by subjects' parents, there was a significant main effect for assessment occasion, $F(1, 165) = 55.40$, $p < .001$; however, neither the group effect, $F(1, 165) < 1$, nor the interaction effect, $F(1, 165) < 1$, was significant (see Table 5.2). Both the childbearing subjects, $t(169) = -5.82$, $p < .001$, and the nonchildbearing subjects, $t(172) = -5.78$, $p < .001$, reported significantly less social support from their parents at 9 weeks postpartum relative to the second trimester of pregnancy.

For support provided by subjects' partners, there was a main effect for occasion, $F(1, 145) = 22.70$, $p < .001$, and the interaction effect was significant, $F(1, 145) = 11.25$, $p < .01$ (see Table 5.2). The main effect for group was not significant, $F(1, 145) < 1$. Paired t-tests revealed that childbearing subjects relative to nonchildbearing subjects reported less support from their partners at 9 weeks postpartum, $t(148) = 2.07$, $p < .05$. Also, the childbearing subjects reported significantly less social support from their spouses at 9 weeks postpartum relative to the second trimester of pregnancy, $t(161) = -4.29$, $p < .001$. Finally, 1 item in the SSI interview administered during pregnancy asked specifically about how much the woman expected her partner to help with childcare after the baby was born. The same item in the postpartum SSI interview asked about how much help the woman was receiving from her partner with childcare. There was a very large difference between what childbearing women expected and what they reported receiving (much less than expected) with respect to help from their partners with childcare, $t(160) = -3.63$, $p < .001$.

An additional measure of social support, the Postpartum Social Support Questionnaire, was administered only to the childbearing subjects. The actual (as perceived by the subject) and desired amount of social support provided by the woman's partner, parents, in-laws, other relatives, and friends is assessed by the PSSQ. Table 5.3 shows the actual and desired levels of support provided by each of the groups of support providers and indicates that each of these groups provided significantly less support than was desired by the childbearing women during the postpartum period.

TABLE 5.2. Means and standard deviations for the confidant, parent, and partner scales of the Social Support Interview during pregnancy and after delivery.

	Social network member		
Group	Confidant	Parent	Partner
	Second trimester		
Childbearing			
M	1.84	2.09	1.47
SD	.51	.68	.47
Nonchildbearing			
M	1.74	2.04	1.55
SD	.46	.69	.50
	9 weeks postpartum		
Childbearing			
M	2.27	2.37	1.68
SD	.68	.81	.52
Nonchildbearing			
M	2.10	2.31	1.57
SD	.67	.85	.49

Note: Higher scores represent lower levels of support.

TABLE 5.3. Paired t-tests of differences between childbearing subjects' actual and desired levels of postpartum support assessed by the Postpartum Social Support Questionnaire.

Source of support	Actual level	Desired level	*t*	*df*
Partner				
M	4.28	5.16	−18.36*	153
SD	.89	.66		
Parents				
M	3.38	4.21	−12.02*	171
SD	1.23	1.14		
Parents-in-law				
M	2.51	3.24	−9.27*	167
SD	1.23	1.49		
Other relatives				
M	2.57	3.52	−13.64*	174
SD	1.14	1.19		
Friends				
M	3.81	4.55	−12.32*	172
SD	1.20	.94		

*$p < .001$
Note: Higher scores represent higher actual and desired levels of support.

Life Events

The total number (positive and negative) of life events and the number of negative life events from the PLES were calculated for the first, second, and third trimesters and the first 9 weeks postpartum. For the total number of life events, there was a main effect for assessment occasion, Exact $F(3, 174) = 16.43, p < .001$; the main effect for group, $F(1, 176) < 1$, and the interaction effect, Exact $F(3, 174) < 1$, were not significant. The general pattern was that the number of total life events was higher in the first trimester and the first 9 weeks postpartum relative to the second and third trimesters (see Table 5.4).

For the number of negative life events throughout pregnancy and the postpartum period, there was a main effect for group, $F(1, 176) = 5.50, p < .05$, and a main effect for assessment occasion, Exact $F(3, 174) = 9.62, p < .001$; however, the interaction effect was not significant, Exact $F(3, 174) < 1$. Childbearing subjects experienced a significantly greater number of negative life events than nonchildbearing subjects during the 9-week postpartum period, $t(176) = 2.24, p < .05$ (see Table 5.4).

The mean score on the Peripartum Events Scale was 6.04 ($SD = 3.07$). This score compared to a mean score of 4.48 ($SD = 3.24$) from a sample of 98 women in an earlier study (O'Hara et al., 1986) recruited from the same setting. The mean number of events occurring during pregnancy, labor, and delivery (excluding pre-existing conditions—subscales 1 to 3) was 5.06 (SD = 2.73). The comparable score from our earlier study was

TABLE 5.4. Means and standard deviations of stressful life events during pregnancy and after delivery.

	Trimester of event occurrence			
Group	First	Second	Third	Postpartum
	Total number of life events			
Childbearing				
M	2.12	1.43	1.31	2.03
SD	1.89	1.77	1.64	1.80
Nonchildbearing				
M	2.18	1.43	1.28	1.85
SD	2.00	1.64	1.62	2.06
	Number of negative life events			
Childbearing				
M	.82	.60	.49	.93
SD	1.20	1.02	1.00	1.35
Nonchildbearing				
M	.73	.45	.43	.64
SD	1.00	.84	.89	1.06

3.54 (SD = 3.15). The percentage of subjects experiencing at least 1 event from each of the subscale domains and the means and standard deviations for each domain are presented in Table 5.5.

The Childcare Stress Inventory contained a list of 20 stressful events that might occur to a woman during the first several weeks after delivery. Subjects indicate which events occurred and then rate the degree (0 to 100) to which each event that occurred was distressing. Table 5.6 presents the percentage of subjects who experienced each event and the mean distress rating for those subjects who experienced the event. The most commonly occurring event (59.3% of subjects) was "House more disorganized than usual." However, its mean distress rating was lowest of all

TABLE 5.5. Means and standard deviations of Peripartum Events Scale subscales and percentage of subjects experiencing at least 1 event for each subscale.

Subscale	Mean	*SD*	% Experiencing at least 1 event
Demographics	.20	.46	18.1
Past obstetric history	.41	.81	26.6
Medical risk factors	.36	.64	28.8
Obstetric risk factors	.45	.66	36.7
Indication for admission to labor and delivery	.27	.46	26.6
Progress in labor	.23	.42	23.2
Method of delivery	.38	.65	29.4
Duration of labor	.25	.46	24.3
Fetal monitoring	2.30	.81	96.0
Delivery complications	.47	.69	36.2
Infant outcome	.70	1.04	45.2

TABLE 5.6. Percentage of childbearing subjects experiencing each event from the Childcare Stress Inventory and means and standard deviations of distress rating for each event.

Type of events	% experiencing event	Distress ratings Mean	*SD*
Labor and/or delivery did not go as hoped	36.3	52.58	31.14
Negative experience at hospital	20.9	53.92	34.19
Conflict over childcare with family or friends	17.6	43.00	26.31
Strain in relationship with husband	26.9	47.14	25.52
Can't give enough time to husband	41.8	46.01	23.93
Not receiving enough attention from husband	28.6	49.65	27.64
Husband doesn't help enough with work	35.7	47.00	24.27
Overwhelmed by demands of infant care	25.3	53.35	30.52
House more disorganized than usual	59.3	40.08	28.08
Problems feeding baby	16.5	55.33	28.10
Can't quiet baby's cries	20.3	49.68	26.03
Can't relax with baby	4.4	43.25	34.15
Baby has health problems	13.2	62.17	35.11
Taking longer than expected to learn to love baby	7.1	37.38	27.85
Trouble establishing regular feeding times	36.3	39.44	26.23
Trouble establishing regular nap and bed times for baby	40.1	45.53	29.32
Don't know what baby needs when crying	17.6	41.41	25.12
Baby rarely seems content	6.0	59.09	27.64
Feel trapped or confined	34.6	43.73	26.61
Miss previous activities or work	33.5	43.43	25.78

of the events. The event with the highest distress rating, not surprisingly, was "Baby has health problems." It was experienced by 13.2% of subjects.

Comparisons of Postpartum Depressed Childbearing and Nonchildbearing Subjects

Postpartum-depressed childbearing and nonchildbearing subjects were compared with respect to our indices of social adjustment, social support, and negative life events across pregnancy and the puerperium. We expected that depressed childbearing subjects would have experienced significantly poorer adjustments in their relationships with their partners, less social support from their partners, and more stressful life events than depressed nonchildbearing subjects.

With respect to social adjustment in postpartum-depressed childbearing and nonchildbearing subjects for the total SAS-SR, neither the effect for group, $F(1, 27) = 2.20$, nor the effect for assessment occasion was significant, Exact $F(4, 24) < 1$. There was a significant interaction, Exact

$F(4, 24) = 2.88$, $p < .05$. However, there were no significant differences between the childbearing and nonchildbearing women at any of the 5 assessments. The pattern showed that the childbearing women reported levels of social maladjustment very similar to the nonchildbearing women except at the 3-week postpartum assessment (see Figure 5.6).

Neither the friends subscale nor the family relationship subscale of the SAS-SR showed any significant effects. The subscale reflecting marital adjustment showed a significant effect for group, $F(1, 24) = 7.29$, $p < .05$. Postpartum-depressed childbearing women showed significantly higher levels of marital maladjustment only at the 9-week postpartum assessment, $t(26) = 2.85$, $p < .01$, and the 6-month postpartum assessment, $t(18.5) = 2.35$, $p < .05$ (see Figure 5.7). There were, however, no significant effects for the Dyadic Adjustment Scale. Finally, with respect to social adjustment, there were no significant effects for the work in home subscale of the SAS-SR.

We also compared depressed childbearing and nonchildbearing subjects on the pre- and postpartum indices of social support from confidants,

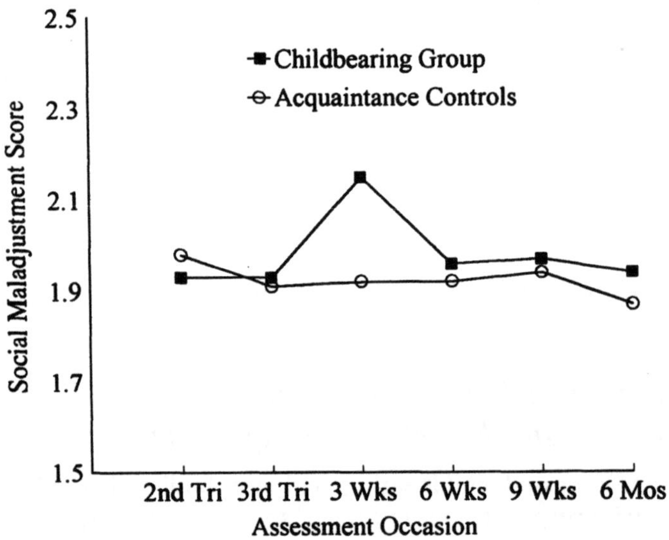

FIGURE 5.6. Total scores on the Social Adjustment Scale-self-report (SAS-SR) for depressed childbearing and nonchildbearing subjects during pregnancy and after delivery. (2nd Tri = second trimester of pregnancy; 3rd Tri = third trimester, 3 Wks = 3 weeks postpartum; 6 Wks = 6 weeks postpartum; 9 Wks = 9 weeks postpartum; 6 Mos = 6 months postpartum.) From "Controlled prospective study of postpartum mood disorders: Comparison of childbearing and nonchildbearing women" by M.W. O'Hara, E.M. Zekoski, L.H. Philipps, & E.J. Wright, 1990, *Journal of Abnormal Psychology, 99,* 3–15. Copyright 1990 by the American Psychological Association. Reprinted by permission of the publisher.

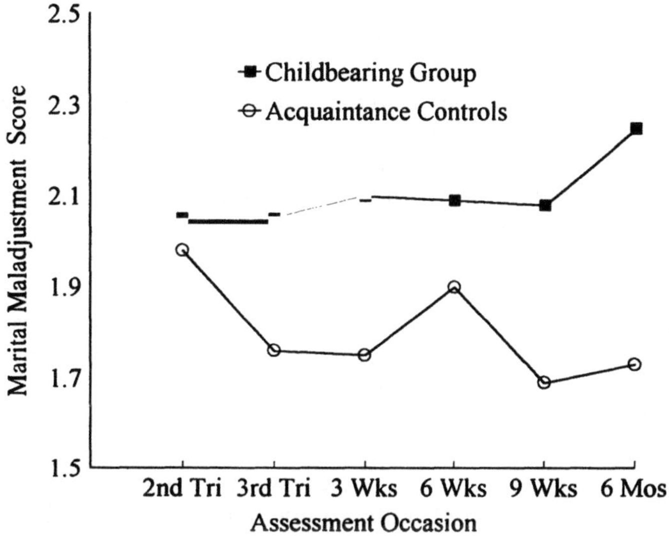

FIGURE 5.7. Scores on the marital adjustment subscale of the Social Adjustment Scale-self-report (SAS-SR) for depressed childbearing and nonchildbearing subjects during pregnancy and after delivery. (2nd Tri = second trimester of pregnancy; 3rd Tri = third trimester; 3 Wks = 3 weeks postpartum; 6 Wks = 6 weeks postpartum; 9 Wks = 9 weeks postpartum; 6 Mos = 6 months postpartum.)

parents, and partners and negative life events from the beginning of pregnancy through the puerperium. There were no differences between the depressed childbearing and nonchildbearing subjects on any of these variables.

Summary

Childbearing subjects showed poorer social adjustment than nonchildbearing subjects early in the postpartum period. Marital adjustment, in particular, was poorer for childbearing subjects beginning in the third trimester and continuing on through the 6-month follow-up assessment. With respect to social support, both childbearing and nonchildbearing subjects reported that social support from their confidants, parents, and partners decreased over the course of the study. Childbearing subjects relative to nonchildbearing subjects reported significantly less social support from their partners and confidants during the postpartum period. Childbearing subjects also expressed general dissatisfaction with the amount of social support they received during the postpartum period. In addition, childbearing subjects reported a greater number of negative life events during the postpartum period than did the nonchildbearing subjects. Finally, there were very few differences between depressed childbearing and depressed nonchildbearing subjects with respect to their social adjustments, social support, and experience of negative life events.

Taking social adjustment as a whole, the early postpartum period (up to 6 to 8 weeks postpartum) was the time when childbearing women showed the poorest social adjustment relative to nonchildbearing women. This finding is not entirely surprising, given that women are typically preoccupied with managing the care of a newborn during this period. To some degree poorer functioning in roles other than that of a mother of a newborn reflects the redirecting of attention and energy from other roles and relationships. Although this process, which is probably necessary and evidently time-limited, is rather normal and adaptive for the mother and child, the woman's partner and other children (if any) may not view it in this way. The conflict that a woman experiences when the demands of household responsibilities and the demands of other family members interfere with her efforts to nurture her newborn, and perhaps even get much-needed rest, may contribute to the anger or irritability that is indicative (on the SAS-SR) of less than optimal functioning in each of the role domains (e.g., family or marital relationship).

The social relationship in which the poorest adjustment occurred according to the SAS-SR, particularly after delivery, was the marital relationship. Differences in marital adjustment between childbearing and nonchildbearing women were not apparent in the second-trimester assessment; however, they emerged by the third trimester and were still evident at 6 months postpartum. Moreover, marital satisfaction, measured by the Dyadic Adjustment Scale, was significantly higher in childbearing women than nonchildbearing women in the second trimester; however, this significant difference disappeared by 9 weeks postpartum. These findings suggest that rather enduring changes occur in the marital relationship of childbearing women.

As was suggested above, the introduction of a new household member and the woman's need to care for the baby may reduce the time that a woman has to give to her partner. The partner may feel left out or abandoned and become irritable and angry himself. Another source of marital dissatisfaction after childbirth is violated expectations. The woman's partner may provide much less help with childcare and household chores than she expected. In fact, the woman may be carrying out all of her normal responsibilities in addition to those associated with caring for the new baby. If proper adjustments are not made in household routines and responsibilities, this source of dissatisfaction could persist over a long period of time. The results from the social support assessment are consistent with this interpretation.

Childbearing subjects reported that they received less social support from and provided less social support to their partners than did nonchildbearing subjects at 9 weeks postpartum; there were no differences in the second trimester. Childbearing subjects also reported a significant decline in the amount of support they received from and provided to their spouses from the second trimester to 9 weeks postpartum. Moreover, the results also indicated that childbearing women received less help with childcare after delivery than they expected (based on an assessment during pregnancy). Finally, childbearing women reported, in the context of the PSSQ, that they received significantly less support from their partners (and other members of their social network) after delivery than they desired. These findings paint a relatively clear picture of dissatisfaction on the part of childbearing women with the support provided after delivery by their partners and, to a lesser extent, by other members (e.g., friends and parents) of their social networks.

Childbearing women experienced a higher level of negative life events than nonchildbearing women, particularly in the first 9 weeks postpartum. There are two major implications of this finding. First, negative life events will have direct effects on the new mother, increasing the likelihood of depression and impairing her ability to cope. Second, these events will also stress other members of the family, increasing the demands on the woman to provide support and assistance to her partner and other children. In total, the new mother must not only manage all of the responsibilities inherent in caring for a new baby but often must cope with unforeseen negative life events as well. These circumstances make it especially important that the family, especially the couple, is prepared for the changes in relationships that will occur after the baby is born and make preparations to cope with these changes in a way that will maximize the mother's social adjustment and that of her entire family.

6
Depression During Pregnancy

Despite the common belief that there is a low incidence of psychiatric disorders during pregnancy (McGrath, Keita, Strickland, & Russo, 1990), we found in both our earlier and current works that the rate of depression during pregnancy was not significantly lower than the rate of depression during the puerperium (O'Hara et al., 1984); see chapter 4. Moreover, chapters 4 and 5 made it clear that childbearing women experience higher levels of depressive symptomatology and lower levels of social adjustment during pregnancy than nonchildbearing women. Interestingly, Elliott et al. (1983) found little evidence of significant mood changes during pregnancy; however, their comparisons were to the norms of the various instruments rather than to the responses of a sample of nonchildbearing women followed prospectively.

Our goal in this part of the research was to test hypotheses regarding the role of psychological and environmental risk factors for depression during pregnancy. We found in our earlier study that depression during pregnancy appeared to be somewhat atypical (O'Hara, 1986). For example, depression during pregnancy was not associated with an increased number of stressful life events, a greater personal or family history of depression, or widespread complaints about lack of social support, all factors that tended to characterize risk for postpartum depression. The women who experienced depression during pregnancy did tend to have especially high levels of somatic complaints and a greater number of children, suggesting the possibility that they may have felt sick more often and may have been unable to take proper care of themselves because of their responsibilities for their children (O'Hara, 1986). Our current study allowed us the opportunity to attempt to replicate these findings.

As discussed earlier, depression was conceptualized in two ways for this study. First, it was conceptualized as a clinical disorder (APA, 1987). We defined this clinical depression using the Research Diagnostic Criteria for major and minor depression (Spitzer et al., 1978). Clinical depressions are important because they cause suffering and impair the functioning of the afflicted person. Depression was also defined as a continuous variable measured by the Beck Depression Inventory. High levels of depressive symptomatology may reflect high levels of negative affect but not necessarily the presence of a clinical depression (Lewinsohn et al., 1988;

O'Hara et al., 1984; Whiffen, 1988). Several studies have shown that risk factors for clinical depression and high levels of depressive symptomatology differ (Lewinsohn et al., 1988; O'Hara et al., 1984; Whiffen, 1988). For this reason we investigated the association between both psychological and environmental risk factors and clinical depression in the second trimester as well as level of depressive symptomatology in the second and third trimesters of pregnancy.

Tests of the associations between risk factors and depression were done separately for the childbearing and nonchildbearing subjects. The results reported in this chapter are organized by particular risk factor (e.g., personal history of psychopathology, negative life events), within risk factor by depression outcome (i.e., clinical diagnosis, self-report of severity), and within depression outcome by childbearing status (i.e., childbearing and nonchildbearing groups).

Depression was assessed at two points in time during pregnancy. Shortly after subjects were recruited, they completed 2 measures of depressive symptomatology, the Beck Depression Inventory (BDI) and the SCL-90-R depression subscale, along with other self-report measures. Subjects also participated in diagnostic interviews for major or minor depression during the month preceding the interview. In the third trimester, at approximately 34 weeks gestation, subjects completed the BDI and the SCL-90-R depression subscale. Because the findings for the BDI and the SCL-90-R depression subscale were largely redundant, only the findings for the BDI will be reported.

Sociodemographic Factors

Depression Diagnosis

The spouses of depressed childbearing subjects had a significantly lower level of educational attainment than the spouses of nondepressed childbearing subjects, $t(172) = -1.98, p < .05$. Also, fewer depressed (35.7%) than nondepressed (68.4%) childbearing subjects were working during pregnancy, $\chi^2(N = 188; 1) = 4.79, p < .05$). Finally, depressed childbearing subjects had a lower socioeconomic status than nondepressed childbearing subjects, $t(186) = -2.94, p < .01$. Variables that did not differentiate depressed and nondepressed childbearing subjects included age, education level, years of marriage, income, previous miscarriage or abortion, number of children, husband's age, education or employment status, private or clinic patient status, religion, and past loss of mother or father.

The only sociodemographic variable to differentiate the depressed and nondepressed nonchildbearing subjects was religion. The depressed nonchildbearing subjects (27.3%) were less likely to be Catholic or Protestant than the nondepressed nonchildbearing subjects (67.8%), $\chi^2(N = 185; 6) = 28.98, p < .001$.

Depressive Symptomatology

Among childbearing subjects at the time of the second-trimester interview, lower education level ($r = -.23$), lower spouse education level ($r = -.29$), lower socioeconomic status ($r = -.34$), not being married, $t(41.8) = -2.38, p < .05$, and being seen as a clinic patient (vs. a private patient), $t(186) = 2.65, p < .01$, were all associated with higher levels of depressive symptomatology. Lower education level ($r = -.20$), lower level of spouse education ($r = -.25$), and lower socioeconomic status ($r = -.15$) were associated with level of depressive symptomatology in the third trimester.

Among nonchildbearing subjects at the time of the second-trimester interview, lower education level ($r = -.17$), lower spouse education level ($r = -.21$), lower socioeconomic level ($r = -.16$), and being unemployed, $t(182) = -2.65, p < .01$, were all associated with higher levels of depressive symptomatology. Lower age ($r = -.25$), lower education level ($r = -.27$), lower level of spouse education ($r = -.28$), and lower socioeconomic status ($r = -.27$) were associated with level of depressive symptomatology in the third trimester.

Personal and Family History of Psychopathology

Depression Diagnosis

Depressed childbearing subjects relative to nondepressed childbearing subjects were significantly more likely to have experienced a previous major depression and premenstrual major depression syndrome (Endicott et al., 1981) and to have had a lifetime diagnosis of alcoholism than nondepressed childbearing subjects (see Table 6.1). A somewhat similar pattern was observed for the nonchildbearing subjects. Depressed nonchildbearing subjects relative to nondepressed nonchildbearing subjects were significantly more likely to have experienced a previous major depression and premenstrual major depression syndrome than nondepressed childbearing subjects and to have a lifetime diagnosis of dysthymia. Finally, depressed nonchildbearing subjects were significantly more likely than the nondepressed nonchildbearing subjects to have spouses with a lifetime diagnosis of alcoholism (see Table 6.2).

Depressive Symptomatology

Among childbearing subjects at the time of the second-trimester interview, previous major depression, $t(184) = 2.52, p < .05$, lifetime pre-

TABLE 6.1. Personal and family history of psychopathology in childbearing depressed and nondepressed subjects.

Variable	Depressed (N = 14) (%)	Nondepressed (N = 174) (%)	χ^2
Past depression	64.3	34.3	5.02*
Premenstrual major depression	64.3	26.4	7.23**
Dysthymia	.0	1.1	<1
Cyclothymia	7.1	1.1	<1
Hypomania	7.1	2.9	<1
Alcoholism	28.6	6.9	5.28*
Generalized anxiety	14.3	2.9	2.06
Depressed first-degree relative	42.9	37.4	<1
Depressed partner	14.3	11.5	<1
Partner with alcohol problem	21.4	10.9	<1

*$p < .05$
**$p < .01$
Note: The total N for these analyses is 188 because some subjects who dropped out prior to the postpartum interview are included. All indices except premenstrual major depression were derived from the second-trimester interview. Premenstrual major depression was derived from the Premenstrual Assessment Form (Halbreich et al., 1982).

menstrual major depression, $t(73.3) = 4.05$, $p < .001$, cyclothymia, $t(186) = 2.01$, $p < .05$, and lifetime history of alcoholism in spouse, $t(22.4) = 2.53$, $p < .05$, were associated with higher levels of depressive symptomatology. Previous major depression, $t(178) = 3.22$, $p < .01$, lifetime

TABLE 6.2. Personal and family history of psychopathology in nonchildbearing depressed and nondepressed subjects.

Variable	Depressed (N = 11) (%)	Nondepressed (N = 175) (%)	χ^2
Past depression	80.0	39.9	4.70*
Premenstrual major depression	54.5	20.0	5.32**
Dysthymia	45.4	1.1	44.54**
Cyclothymia	9.1	3.4	<1
Hypomania	18.2	5.7	<1
Alcoholism	18.2	8.0	<1
Generalized anxiety	9.1	7.4	<1
Depressed first-degree relative	36.4	38.9	<1
Depressed partner	18.2	9.7	<1
Partner with alcohol problem	36.4	8.0	6.56*

*$p < .05$
**$p < .01$
Note: The total N for these analyses is 186 because some subjects who dropped out prior to the postpartum interview are included. All indices except premenstrual major depression were derived from the second-trimester interview. Premenstrual major depression was derived from the Premenstrual Assessment Form (Halbreich et al., 1982).

history of premenstrual major depression, $t(180) = 3.15$, $p < .01$, lifetime history of depression in a first-degree relative, $t(180) = 2.01$, $p < .05$, lifetime history of alcoholism, $t(180) = 2.03$, $p < .05$, and lifetime history of alcoholism in spouse, $t(22.0) = 2.59$, $p < .05$, were all associated with higher levels of depressive symptomatology in the third trimester.

Among nonchildbearing subjects at the time of the second-trimester interview, previous major depression, $t(179) = 2.62$, $p < .05$, and lifetime premenstrual major depression, $t(182) = 6.18$, $p < .001$, cyclothymia, $t(182) = 2.19$, $p < .05$, and alcoholism, $t(182) = 3.00$, $p < .01$, were associated with higher levels of depressive symptomatology. Previous major depression, $t(114.5) = 2.95$, $p < .01$, lifetime history of premenstrual major depression, $t(44.3) = 4.85$, $p < .001$, and alcoholism, $t(176) = 2.05$, $p < .05$, were all associated with higher levels of depressive symptomatology in the third trimester.

Social Support During Pregnancy

Depression Diagnosis

Social support provided by the subjects' closest confidants, parents, and partners was assessed in the Social Support Interview. Among the childbearing women, there were no differences between the depressed and nondepressed subjects with respect to social support from the women's confidants and parents. Depressed women, however, did report a lower level of support from their partners than did nondepressed women, $t(13.9) = 2.21$, $p < .05$. Depressed women also reported less overall satisfaction with the support that they had been receiving than nondepressed women, $t(13.8) = 2.51$, $p < .05$. Among the nonchildbearing women, depressed subjects reported significantly more social support from their confidants than nondepressed subjects, $t(13.8) = -3.29$, $p < .01$. There were no differences between depressed and nondepressed nonchildbearing subjects with respect to support from parents or partners or satisfaction with overall support.

Depressive Symptomatology

Among childbearing subjects at the time of the second-trimester interview, there were significant associations between level of depressive symptomatology and social support from the parents ($r = .21$), and partners ($r = .24$), and overall satisfaction with support ($r = .22$). Among childbearing subjects in the third trimester, there were significant associations between the level of depressive symptomatology and social support received from the parents ($r = .16$) and partners ($r = .17$), and overall satisfaction with support ($r = .22$).

Among the nonchildbearing subjects at the time of the second-trimester interview, only support provided by the partner ($r = .27$) and overall satisfaction with support ($r = .21$) were related to level of depressive symptomatology. In the third trimester, only support provided by the partner ($r = .24$) and overall satisfaction with support ($r = .18$) were associated with level of depressive symptomatology.

Negative Life Events

Depression Diagnosis

Measures of the number of negative life events for the first and second trimesters of pregnancy were obtained (see Table 6.3). The depressed childbearing subjects reported experiencing significantly more negative life events than nondepressed childbearing subjects during the second trimester of pregnancy, $t(184) = 3.25, p < .01$. Depressed nonchildbearing subjects reported significantly higher levels of negative life events in the first trimester than nondepressed nonchildbearing subjects, $t(183) = 2.38$, $p < .05$.

Depressive Symptomatology

Among childbearing subjects higher levels of negative life events during the second trimester were associated with higher levels of depressive

TABLE 6.3. Means and standard deviations of negative life events during the first and second trimesters of pregnancy among depressed and nondepressed childbearing and nonchildbearing subjects.

	Depression status	
Group	Depressed	Nondepressed
	First trimester	
Childbearing		
M	1.36	.79
SD	1.95	1.12
Nonchildbearing		
M	1.45	.70
SD	1.29	1.00
	Second trimester	
Childbearing	1.43	.53
M	1.16	.98
SD		
Nonchildbearing		
M	1.36	.43
SD	1.69	.76

symptomatology during the second (r = .27) and third trimesters (r = .21). Among the nonchildbearing subjects, there was a significant association between level of depressive symptomatology in the second trimester and number of negative life events in the first (r = .15) and second (r = .16) trimesters.

Social Adjustment

Depression Diagnosis

Overall, the depressed childbearing subjects reported lower levels of social adjustment on the Social Adjustment Scale-self-report (SAS-SR) than the nondepressed childbearing subjects at the time of the second-trimester assessment and in the third trimester. For example, in the second trimester, relative to nondepressed childbearing subjects, the depressed childbearing subjects reported poorer (1) overall adjustment, $t(186) = 4.69, p < .001$; (2) marital adjustment, $t(12.75) = 2.24, p < .05$; (3) adjustment in relationship with friends, $t(13.89) = 2.74, p < .05$; and (4) adjustment in work at home, $t(186) = 3.05, p < .01$. Marital adjustment as assessed by the Dyadic Adjustment Scale did not differentiate the depressed and nondepressed childbearing subjects. A similar pattern was observed for social adjustment assessed in the third trimester. The depressed childbearing subjects relative to the nondepressed childbearing subjects reported poorer (1) overall adjustment, $t(180) = 4.99, p < .001$; (2) marital adjustment, $t(162) = 2.99, p < .01$; (3) adjustment in relationship with friends, $t(180) = 3.21, p < .01$; and (4) adjustment in work at home, $t(179) = 3.19, p < .01$.

In the second trimester, the depressed nonchildbearing subjects relative to the nondepressed nonchildbearing subjects reported poorer (1) overall adjustment, $t(183) = 3.73, p < .001$; and (2) marital adjustment, $t(161) = 3.24, p < .01$. There were no differences between depressed and nondepressed subjects with respect to marital adjustment measured by the DAS. A similar pattern was observed for social adjustment assessed in the third trimester. The depressed nonchildbearing subjects relative to the nondepressed nonchildbearing subjects reported poorer (1) overall adjustment, $t(176) = 2.33, p < .05$; and (2) adjustment in work at home, $t(175) = 2.06, p < .05$.

Depressive Symptomatology

Among childbearing and nonchildbearing subjects at the time of the second-trimester interview, there was a significant association between level of depressive symptomatology and the Social Adjustment Scale-self-report (and most of its subscales) and the Dyadic Adjustment Scale (see Table 6.4). This pattern also was observed for the third-trimester assess-

TABLE 6.4. Association between social and marital adjustment and level of depressive symptomatology among childbearing and nonchildbearing subjects during the second and third trimesters of pregnancy.

Scale	Group	
	Childbearing	Nonchildbearing
	Second-trimester correlations	
SAS-SR		
Marital relationship	.44	.43
Family relationships	.31	.37
Relationship with friends	.50	.36
Work at home	.48	.16
Overall adjustment	.61	.53
Dyadic Adjustment Scale	−.37	−.39
	Third-trimester correlations	
SAS-SR		
Marital relationship	.59	.43
Family relationships	.44	.56
Relationship with friends	.49	.64
Work at home	.57	.50
Overall adjustment	.73	.76
Dyadic Adjustment Scale (second trimester)	−.24	−.29

Note: All correlations are significant, at least $p < .05$.

ments of social adjustment and depressive symptomatology for both childbearing and nonchildbearing subjects (see Table 6.4).

Cognitive Constructs

The Self-Control Questionnaire was obtained in the second trimester. Depressed childbearing subjects relative to nondepressed childbearing subjects showed more dysfunctional self-control attitudes, $t(186) = 2.81$, $p < .01$. The same findings were obtained for depressed and nondepressed nonchildbearing subjects, $t(182) = 2.66$, $p < .01$. Among both childbearing and nonchildbearing subjects, there were significant associations between self-control attitudes and levels of depressive symptomatology in the second and third trimesters (see Table 6.5).

Summary

Depressed childbearing women relative to nondepressed childbearing women tended to have lower socioeconomic status, histories of past depression and alcoholism, less support from their partners, more negative life events, poorer social adjustment, and more dysfunctional self-

TABLE 6.5. Association between self-control attitudes during the second trimester of pregnancy and level of depressive symptomatology among childbearing and nonchildbearing subjects during the second the third trimesters of pregnancy.

Times of depression assessment	Group	
	Childbearing	Nonchildbearing
Second trimester	.28	.18
Third trimester	.27	.16

Note: All correlations are significant, at least $p < .05$.

control attitudes. The findings regarding the association of depression risk factors and level of depressive symptomatology in the second and third trimesters were similar and somewhat more consistent. For example, several indices of lower SES (e.g., lower personal and spouse education, unmarried, being seen as clinic patient) and history of personal and family psychopathology (e.g., major depression, premenstrual major depression, alcoholism, alcoholism in spouse) were significantly associated with level of depressive symptomatology during pregnancy.

The findings of our previous study suggested that traditional risk factors for depression would not emerge as significant predictors of depression during pregnancy (O'Hara, 1986). However, the results of this study suggested just the opposite—all of the classic risk factors were found to be associated with depression during pregnancy. It is not easy to account for the different results of the two studies, given that subjects were recruited from the same setting and the study methods were similar (with the exception of the control group in the current study).

The findings for the childbearing subjects did share much in common with earlier studies that have evaluated risk factors for high levels of depressive symptomatology or clinical depression during pregnancy. Several studies have found that indices of lower SES are associated with higher levels of depression during pregnancy (Cox et al., 1982; Gotlib et al., 1989; Zajicek, 1981). Perhaps related findings are that higher levels of stressful life events have been found to be associated with depression during pregnancy (Martin, Brown, Goldberg, & Brockington, 1989; Zajicek, 1981) and that women experiencing marital problems are more likely to have higher levels of depression during pregnancy (Kumar & Robson, 1984). All of these findings suggest that social stress may play an important role in accounting for both clinical depression and high levels of negative affect. It is easy to imagine that these social stress factors (i.e., few financial resources, little spouse support) combined with the prospects of managing a new baby would be depressogenic.

Relatively few studies have examined past psychiatric history as a risk factor for depression during pregnancy; however, there has been some evidence to suggest that women with a history of depression are vulnerable to depression during pregnancy (Kumar & Robson, 1984; Wolkind, 1974; Zajicek, 1981), one of our earlier studies being the major exception (O'Hara, 1986). These findings and findings that were earlier described (see Chapter 2) and will be described (see Chapter 8) point to the importance of continuing or rather stable risk for depression throughout the childbearing years. For example, several studies have demonstrated that past depression predicts postpartum depression and that postpartum depression puts a woman at risk for recurrence of depression in future years (O'Hara et al., 1983; Philipps & O'Hara, 1991). These findings have implications for the care of childbearing-age women by health and mental health professionals. These implications will be discussed in chapter 9.

The findings for the comparisons of depressed and nondepressed nonchildbearing women were similar to, if not quite so robust as, the findings for the depressed and nondepressed childbearing women. For example, there was no evidence of lower SES among the depressed nonchildbearing women (based on RDC), nor was there any evidence of significantly lower levels of social support for these women. Moreover, the higher level of negative life events observed during pregnancy for the depressed nonchildbearing women was evident in the first trimester but not in the second trimester, as was the case for the depressed childbearing subjects. The only major risk factor that was really salient for the depressed nonchildbearing women was past history of depression (including premenstrual depression and dysthymia). The relatively few risk factors associated with depression in the nonchildbearing women at the "pregnancy" assessment is similar to the case for postpartum depression. The most theoretically plausible explanation is that the stress of pregnancy interacts with other risk or vulnerability factors to increase the likelihood that these factors (e.g., negative life events, poor spousal support) will show significant associations with the presence of clinical depression during pregnancy.

For nonchildbearing subjects there was a moderate degree of association between the depression risk and vulnerability factors and levels of depressive symptomatology during the second and third trimesters. The specific significant associations and their strengths were relatively similar for the nonchildbearing and childbearing subjects. These findings would suggest that risk factors affecting depressive symptomatology in childbearing subjects are not particularly unique to pregnancy even though levels of depressive symptomatology are higher in childbearing subjects than in nonchildbearing subjects during the second and third trimesters of pregnancy.

The findings regarding the psychological adjustment of childbearing and nonchildbearing women during pregnancy do suggest that although there were no differences in the rates of RDC-defined depression, there was some evidence that a wider variety of risk factors were significantly associated with depression in childbearing than nonchildbearing women. In contrast to the rates of clinical depression, there was good evidence that childbearing women experience higher levels of depressive symptomatology and poorer social adjustment during pregnancy than nonchildbearing women. Nevertheless, the range of risk factors significantly associated with depressive symptomatology during pregnancy is similar for both childbearing and nonchildbearing groups. Although our findings suggested that childbearing and nonchildbearing women may be relatively comparable throughout pregnancy, the experiences of labor, delivery, and the early puerperium certainly are radically different from those of nonchildbearing women. It is during this period that the postpartum blues emerge, and it is this issue that will be discussed next.

7
Postpartum Blues

Many of our childbearing subjects experienced the blues after delivery. As we described in chapter 4, between 26% and 42% of childbearing subjects experienced the blues as compared to between 7% and 10% of nonchildbearing subjects who experienced blues-like symptoms. The lower and upper bounds of prevalence rates reflected the use of two sets of criteria, the Handley and Pitt criteria, respectively (O'Hara et al., 1990). Two different sets of criteria were used to define the postpartum blues because there is no accepted set of criteria for the blues (Kennerley & Gath, 1989a; O'Hara, 1991). What is accepted is that the blues are usually of brief duration and that they begin sometime in the first week to 10 days after delivery.

Unlike the case for prepartum and postpartum depression, there was a major difference in the rate of the blues across childbearing and nonchildbearing subjects. The pattern of the blues symptoms in the childbearing subjects was also very distinctive relative to the pattern of the blues symptoms in the nonchildbearing subjects (i.e., the clear peaking of symptoms on days 4 to 8 postpartum vs. no peaking for nonchildbearing women). For these reasons this chapter will address potential causal factors of the blues in childbearing women only.

Several sets of variables, identified in previous studies as possibly causing or at least increasing a woman's risk for the blues or depression, were studied. Although there was not strong support in the literature, several sociodemographic variables were also included in the study. For example, variables such as younger age, lower socioeconomic status, and primiparity could be viewed as markers for a relative lack of preparedness for childbearing in an emotional, economic, or practical sense. Other risk factors that we investigated with respect to the blues included psychiatric history variables, marital and social adjustment during pregnancy, social support during pregnancy, stressful life events during pregnancy and immediately after delivery, and hormonal factors.

Both the Handley and the Pitt blues classifications were made retrospectively during the 9-week postpartum interview. Although the number of women identified by each set of criteria were different, both determinations were made at the same time, using roughly the same method. Of the two sets of criteria, we selected the Handley criteria to serve as our main retrospective index of the blues (O'Hara, Schlechte, Lewis, & Wright, 1991). To complement the retrospective index, we created a second index based on the postpartum VAS ratings made by all participants. This second index was designed as a self-report measure that was obtained contemporaneously with the postpartum period under consideration (first week postpartum). The characteristics of this measure are described next.

Classification of the Blues

A VAS-based blues classification (VAS Blues) was created on the basis of the peak observed the VAS across days 4, 6, and 8 for the entire sample of childbearing women (O'Hara et al., 1990). The mean VAS score for those 3 days (the last 3 VAS assessments) was calculated for each subject. Subjects whose scores were among the highest 26% were included in the VAS Blues group (Mean VAS = 50.06, SD = 6.58); all other subjects were included in the VAS Non-Blues group (Mean VAS = 25.66, SD = 8.59). The 26% cutoff was used because it corresponded to the proportion of subjects meeting Handley criteria for the blues (O'Hara et al., 1990). There were no points of rarity that provided a more sensible blues cutoff on the mean VAS for days 4, 6, and 8.

There was a 74.6% agreement between the Handley and VAS measures of the blues, $\chi^2(1; N = 181) = 20.80$, $p < .001$. In 12.7% of cases, women met Handley Blues criteria but not VAS Blues criteria. Also, in 12.7% of cases, women met VAS Blues criteria but not Handley Blues criteria.

Results

Demographic Risk Factors

There were no differences between women who met criteria for either the Handley Blues or the VAS Blues and women who did not meet blues criteria with respect to age, education, marital status, parity, clinic vs. private patient status, employment status, previous death of mother or father, and husband's age, education, and employment status.

Depression Risk Factors

Depressive Symptomatology During Pregnancy

Women who met the Handley Blues criteria had higher levels of depressive symptomatology as measured by the Beck Depression Inventory during the second trimester of pregnancy than women who did not meet

TABLE 7.1. Means and standard deviations of Beck Depression Inventory scores during the second and third trimesters for subjects meeting and not meeting Handley and VAS Blues criteria.

	Blues criteria			
	Handley		VAS	
Trimester of assessment	Yes ($N = 48$)	No ($N = 134$)	Yes ($N = 47$)	No ($N = 134$)
Second				
M	9.40	7.01	9.87	6.84
SD	6.09	4.73	6.85	4.28
Third				
M	11.34	7.44	10.72	7.68
SD	6.75	4.97	6.29	5.36

the Handley Blues criteria, $t(180) = 2.76$, $p < .01$; the same pattern held for the VAS Blues criteria, $t(59) = 2.85$, $p < .01$ (see Table 7.1). In the third trimester a similar pattern emerged. Both women meeting the Handley Blues criteria, $t(177) = 4.18$, $p < .001$, and women meeting the VAS Blues criteria, $t(176) = 3.16$, $p < .01$, had significantly higher levels of depressive symptomatology than women not meeting blues criteria (see Table 7.1).

DEPRESSION DIAGNOSIS

Neither women who met Handley Blues criteria, $\chi^2(1; N = 182) = 3.14$, n.s., nor women who met VAS Blues criteria, $\chi^2(1; N = 181) = 1.95$, n.s., were more likely to have met the RDC for major or minor depression at the time of the second-trimester interview than women who did not meet blues criteria (see Table 7.2). However, women who met Handley Blues criteria, $\chi^2(1; N = 182) = 10.59$, $p < .01$, and women who met VAS Blues criteria, $\chi^2(1; N = 181) = 16.59$, $p < .001$), were more likely to have had a depression prior to pregnancy than women who did not meet either blues criteria. Also, both women who met Handley Blues criteria, $\chi^2(1; N = 182) = 5.10$, $p < .05$, and women who met VAS Blues criteria, $\chi^2(1; N = 181) = 5.22$, $p < .05$, were more likely to have a lifetime diagnosis of cyclothymia than women who did not meet blues criteria. Both women who met Handley Blues criteria, $\chi^2(1; N = 182) = 7.36$, $p < .01$, and women who met VAS Blues criteria, $\chi^2(1; N = 181) = 5.93$, $p < .05$, were more likely to have met criteria for premenstrual major depression prior to pregnancy than women who did not meet blues criteria. Finally, both women who met Handley Blues criteria, $\chi^2(1; N = 182) = 14.78$, $p < .001$, and women who met the VAS Blues criteria, $\chi^2(1; N = 181) = 7.47$, $p < .01$, were more likely to experience postpartum depression than women who did not meet Blues criteria.

TABLE 7.2. Personal history of psychopathology in women meeting and not meeting Handley and VAS blue criteria.

	Blues criteria			
	Handley		VAS	
Psychopathology variable	Yes (N = 48) %	No (N = 134) %	Yes (N = 47) %	No (N = 134) %
Pregnancy depression	14.6	5.2	12.8	5.2
Postpartum depression	25.0	5.2	21.3	6.0
Past depression	56.2	29.8	61.7	28.4
Premenstrual major depression	43.7	23.1	42.6	23.9
Dysthymia	4.2	.0	2.1	.7
Cyclothymia	6.2	.0	6.4	.0
Hypomania	6.2	2.2	.0	4.5
Alcoholism	12.5	6.7	14.9	6.0
Generalized anxiety	6.2	3.0	4.3	3.7

FAMILY HISTORY OF PSYCHOPATHOLOGY

Both women who met the Handley Blues criteria, $\chi^2(1; N = 182) = 4.69$, $p < .05$, and women who met VAS Blues criteria, $\chi^2(1; N = 181) = 14.29$, $p < .001$, were more likely than women who did not meet blues criteria to have fathers with a lifetime history of depression (see Table 7.3). Women meeting the Handley Blues criteria, $\chi^2(1; N = 182) = 6.98$, $p < .01$, were more likely to have mothers with a lifetime history of depression than women who did not meet Handley Blues criteria. The same pattern did not hold for women meeting the VAS Blues criteria. Finally, women meeting the VAS Blues criteria, $\chi^2(1; N = 181) = 4.70$, $p < .05$, were more likely than women not meeting VAS Blues criteria to have siblings with a lifetime history of depression. The same pattern did not hold for women meeting the Handley Blues criteria.

Social Adjustment During Pregnancy

SECOND TRIMESTER

Women who met the Handley Blues criteria reported lower levels of overall social adjustment on the Social Adjustment Scale-self-report during the second trimester of pregnancy than women who did not meet the Handley Blues criteria, $t(180) = 3.16$, $p < .01$. Similar findings were obtained for relationships with friends, $t(180) = 2.50$, $p < .05$, and relationships with extended families, $t(180) = 4.08$, $p < .001$. A similar pattern held for the VAS Blues criteria. Women who met VAS Blues criteria reported poorer (1) overall social adjustment, $t(179) = 3.53$, $p < .01$); (2) relationship with extended families, $t(179) = 3.21$, $p < .01$; (3) adjustment to household work, $t(179) = 2.85$, $p < .01$; and (4) marital

TABLE 7.3. Family history of psychopathology in women meeting and not meeting Handley and VAS Blues criteria.

	Blues criteria			
	Handley		VAS	
Family history variable	Yes (N = 48) %	No (N = 134) %	Yes (N = 47) %	No (N = 134) %
Depressed sibling	27.1	20.9	34.0	18.7
Depressed mother	25.0	9.7	21.3	11.2
Depressed father	20.8	9.0	27.7	6.7
Depressed partner	18.7	9.7	17.0	10.4
Partner with alcohol problem	18.7	9.0	21.3	8.2

adjustment, $t(163) = 3.24$, $p < .01$, than women who did not experience the blues. With respect to marital adjustment measured by the Dyadic Adjustment Scale, neither women who met Handley Blues criteria nor women who met VAS Blues criteria had lower levels of self-reported marital adjustment during pregnancy than women who did not meet blues criteria (see Table 7.4).

THIRD TRIMESTER

Women who met Handley Blues criteria reported poorer (1) overall social adjustment, $t(177) = 3.23$, $p < .01$; (2) marital adjustment, $t(159) = 2.08$, $p < .05$; and (3) adjustment to household work, $t(176) = 3.08$, $p < .01$, than women who did not meet Handley Blues criteria. Similarly, women who met VAS Blues criteria reported poorer (1) overall social adjustment, $t(176) = 3.78$, $p < .001$; (2) marital adjustment, $t(158) = 2.86$, $p < .01$; (3) relationships with extended families, $t(176) = 2.34$, $p < .05$; (4) relationships with friends, $t(176) = 2.18$, $p < .05$; and (5) adjustment to household work, $t(175) = 2.70$, $p < .01$, than women who did not meet VAS Blues criteria.

Life Events

Women who met the Handley Blues criteria, $t(180) = 2.11$, $p < .05$, experienced more negative life events during the second trimester of pregnancy (but not the first or third trimester) than women who did not meet Handley Blues criteria; the same pattern held for the VAS Blues criteria, $t(179) = 2.94$, $p < .01$. There were no differences between women who met either the Handley Blues criteria or the VAS Blues criteria and women who did not meet criteria for the blues with respect to the number of peripartum stressful events. Women who met the Handley Blues criteria had higher levels of childcare-related stressors than women who did not meet the Handley Blues criteria, $t(180) = 5.35$, $p < .001$; the same pattern held for the VAS Blues criteria, $t(179) = 4.49$, $p < .001$ (see Table 7.5).

TABLE 7.4. Means and standard deviatons of social and marital adjustment scales obtained during the second and third trimesters of pregnancy among women meeting and not meeting Handley and VAS Blues criteria.

	Blues criteria			
	Handley		VAS	
Scale	Yes ($N = 48$)	No ($N = 134$)	Yes ($N = 47$)	No ($N = 134$)
	Second trimester			
SAS-SR				
Marital relationship[1]	1.99	1.88	2.07	1.85
	(.45)	(.39)	(.36)	(.41)
Family relationships	1.73	1.49	1.69	1.50
	(.43)	(.33)	(.39)	(.35)
Relationships with friends	2.20	1.98	2.12	2.00
	(.71)	(.44)	(.50)	(.53)
Work at home	2.00	1.91	2.10	1.87
	(.56)	(.47)	(.49)	(.48)
Overall adjustment	1.95	1.78	1.97	1.78
	(.38)	(.31)	(.32)	(.33)
Dyadic Adjustment Scale	110.87	113.55	109.11	113.91
	(19.17)	(14.46)	(14.84)	(16.26)
	Third Trimester			
SAS-SR				
Marital relationship	2.14	1.96	2.19	1.94
	(.54)	(.47)	(.52)	(.47)
Family relationships	1.59	1.49	1.62	1.48
	(.35)	(.35)	(.40)	(.33)
Relationships with friends	2.05	1.90	2.06	1.89
	(.49)	(.44)	(.47)	(.44)
Work at home	2.08	1.82	2.06	1.83
	(.56)	(.47)	(.58)	(.47)
Overall adjustment	1.93	1.75	1.95	1.74
	(.38)	(.31)	(.37)	(.31)

[1] For Handley criteria, Yes ($N = 48$); No ($N = 120$). For VAS criteria, Yes ($N = 47$); No ($N = 119$).
Note: Standard deviations are in parentheses.

Social Support

There were no differences between women who met Handley Blues criteria and women who did not meet Handley Blues criteria with respect to social support from their confidants, parents, and partners. The same findings were obtained when the VAS Blues criteria were used to define the blues. However, women who met Handley Blues criteria reported significantly less overall satisfaction with the social support they were receiving during pregnancy than women who did not meet Handley Blues criteria, $t(180) = 2.82$, $p < .01$; the same findings were not obtained for

TABLE 7.5. Means and standard deviations of measures of negative life events during pregnancy, the Peripartum Events Schedule, and the Childcare Stress Inventory among women meeting and not meeting Handley and VAS Blues criteria.

	Blues criteria			
	Handley		VAS	
Scale	Yes ($N = 48$)	No ($N = 134$)	Yes ($N = 47$)	No ($N = 134$)
Negative life events				
First trimester	.94	.78	.83	.80
	(1.34)	(1.17)	(1.11)	(1.22)
Second trimester	.87	.51	.98	.48
	(1.14)	(.96)	(1.13)	(0.96)
Third trimester	.60	.46	.68	.43
	(1.12)	(.97)	(1.14)	(.95)
Peripartum Events Scale	6.06	5.19	5.40	5.42
	(3.41)	(2.59)	(2.28)	(3.03)
Childcare Stress Inventory	8.72	5.25	8.40	5.40
	(4.93)	(3.40)	(4.40)	(3.78)

Note: Standard deviations are in parentheses.

the VAS Blues criteria. Finally, women who met VAS Blues criteria relative to women who did not meet VAS Blues criteria reported that they expected less help with childcare after delivery from their parents, $t(173) = 2.62$, $p < .01$, and their partners, $t(166) = 2.61$, $p = .01$.

Hormonal Factors

REPRODUCTIVE HORMONES

Multivariate analyses of variance were conducted for each of the reproductive hormones comparing women who met and those who did not meet the Handley Blues and the VAS Blues criteria. There were no significant effects for the VAS Blues criteria for any of the hormonal variables. However, there were significant effects for the Handley Blues for free estriol, multivariate $F(1, 138) = 3.94$, $p < .05$, and total estriol, multivariate $F(1, 138) = 4.71$, $p < .05$. Women who met Handley criteria for the blues had higher levels of free estriol at week 38 of gestation, $t(152) = 2.63$, $p < .01$, and day 4 postpartum, $t(163) = 2.50$, $p < .05$, and higher levels of total estriol at week 34 of gestation, $t(167) = 2.13$, $p < .05$, week 36 of gestation, $t(163) = 2.22$, $p < .05$, day 2 postpartum, $t(169) = 4.20$, $p < .001$, and day 3 postpartum, $t(168) = 2.78$, $p < .01$ (see Table 7.6). There were no differences between women who met and did not meet the Handley Blues criteria for estradiol, progesterone, and prolactin. Also, there were no significant differences between women who met and did not meet the Handley or the VAS Blues criteria for the

TABLE 7.6. Prepartum and postpartum levels of reproductive hormones for women meeting and not meeting Handley Blues criteria.

	Week of gestation			Postpartum day					
Hormone	34	36	38	1	2	3	4 (A.M.)	6	8
Estradiol (pmol/d)									
Blues									
M	30,845	34,166	36,788	3,651	1,686	681	522	386	337
SD	15,892	20,366	21,427	2,823	1,409	408	327	203	182
Nonblues									
M	29,389	31,843	34,271	3,802	1,740	729	524	382	301
SD	15,470	18,400	19,119	2,958	1,436	463	318	266	162
Total estriol (nmol/d)									
Blues									
M	400	523	681	137	109	47	18	3.6	1.3
SD	159	293	355	100	86	44	22	4.5	1.5
Nonblues									
M	339	425	586	117	61	30	13	2.8	1.7
SD	160	226	325	79	56	30	23	5.3	4.1
Free estriol (nmol/d)									
Blues									
M	48	59	85	4.7	4.0	2.5	1.8	.8	.4
SD	27	31	43	4.3	4.5	2.5	2.0	1.0	.6

Nonblues									
M	43	51	68	4.5	2.8	1.8	1.1	.6	.4
SD	19	24	30	5.3	3.2	2.5	1.3	.8	.6
Progesterone (nmol/L)									
Blues									
M	304	400	369	55	18	9.6	7.3	3.0	2.1
SD	187	326	240	58	15	8.4	4.9	1.8	1.5
Nonblues									
M	311	349	423	44	16	8.7	6.6	2.9	2.2
SD	199	241	290	40	9.8	5.4	4.0	2.0	1.9
Prolactin (μg/L)									
Blues									
M	171	182	193	159	222	177	174	140	128
SD	74	71	69	85	128	101	86	81	85
Nonblues									
M	180	198	214	174	213	170	179	139	135
SD	80	99	100	103	113	81	107	93	148

Note: Sample sizes ranged from 148 to 169; smaller sample sizes usually occurred at week 38 of gestation because some subjects had delivered. From "Prospective study of postpartum blues: Biologic and psychosocial factors" by M. W. O'Hara, J. A. Schlechte, D. A. Lewis, & E. J. Wright, 1991, *Archives of General Psychiatry, 48,* 801–806. Copyright 1991, American Medical Association. Adapted by permission.

ratios of prolactin to estradiol or progesterone for any of the assessment occasions. Free estriol showed a significant drop from the average level of the prepartum assessments to the day 1 postpartum level for women meeting Handley Blues criteria relative to women not meeting Handley Blues criteria, $t(165) = 2.29, p < .05$.

Glucocorticoid Hormones

Multivariate analyses of variance also were conducted for each of the glucocorticoid hormones comparing women who met and women who did not meet the Handley Blues and the VAS Blues criteria. There were no overall differences between women who met and those who did not meet the Handley or the VAS Blues criteria for total cortisol or urinary free cortisol (see Table 7.7). However, women who met Handley criteria for the blues did have significantly lower levels of total cortisol at week 38 of gestation, $t(152) = -2.08, p < .05$. With respect to dexamethasone suppression, nonsuppression was defined as a 7:00 A.M. or 4:00 P.M. post dexamethasone cortisol > 140 nmol/L. As we reported earlier (O'Hara, Schlechte Lewis, & Wright, 1991), overall there was a very high rate of nonsuppression at both the 7:00 A.M. assessment (92.1%) and the 4:00 P.M. assessment (93.8%). There were no differences between women who met either criteria for the blues and women who did not meet blues criteria at either assessment. As we implied above, there were no differences between women who met and those who did not meet either blues criteria in levels of free or total cortisol at either the 7:00 A.M. or 4:00 P.M. post dexamethasone assessments.

Breast-feeding was not associated with the blues defined by either the Handley criteria, $\chi^2(1; N = 169) < 1$, or the VAS criteria, $\chi^2(1; N = 168) = 1.02$ (see Table 7.8), nor was occurrence of caesarean section associated with either index of the blues.

Summary

Women who experienced higher levels of depressive symptomatology and lower levels of social adjustment during the second and third trimesters of pregnancy were at increased risk for the blues. Moreover, women who had a previous history of depression or who had depressed first-degree relatives, particularly fathers, were at increased risk for the blues. Surprisingly, given these findings, women who experienced a major or minor depression during the second trimester of pregnancy were not at increased risk for the blues.

Negative life events during the second trimester of pregnancy but not during the third trimester were related to increased risk for the blues. Also, women who experienced higher levels of childcare-related stressors

TABLE 7.7. Prepartum and postpartum levels of glucocorticoid hormones for women meeting and not meeting Handley Blues criteria.

	Week of gestation			Postpartum day						
Hormone	34	36	38	1	2	3	4 (A.M.)	4 (P.M.)	6	8
Total cortisol (nmol/L)										
Blues										
M	932	900	838	720	714	680	354	458	681	674
SD	290	264	242	265	252	231	241	237	239	205
Nonblues										
M	902	921	928	773	710	694	328	406	746	695
SD	246	251	238	265	762	228	219	199	218	235
Urinary free cortisol (nmol/d)										
Blues										
M	231	235	241		193		125			
SD	117	114	93		102		78			
Nonblues										
M	231	226	230		200		115			
SD	89	82	80		134		104			

Note: Sample sizes ranged from 152 to 173; smaller sample sizes usually occurred at week 38 of gestation because some subjects had delivered.

TABLE 7.8. Percentage of breast-feeding women and women undergoing a caesarean section meeting and not meeting Handley and VAS Blues criteria.

	Blues criteria			
	Handley		VAS	
Variable	Yes (N = 48) %	No (N = 134) %	Yes (N = 47) %	No (N = 134) %
Breast-feeding	78.6	81.1	85.7	78.6
Caesarean section	14.3	15.6	18.6	14.2

after delivery were at increased risk for the blues. However, obstetrical stressors were not associated with risk for the blues. Social support during the second trimester, in the main, was not associated with increased risk for the blues, with a few exceptions. Women who met Handley criteria reported less overall satisfaction with social support during the second trimester than did women not experiencing the blues. Also, women who met VAS criteria for the blues reported expecting less help with childcare after delivery from their parents and partners than did women not meeting blues criteria.

With respect to hormonal variables, only free and total estriol levels showed any association with indices of the blues (higher levels in women experiencing the blues). These findings, in general, were contrary to our prediction of lower estrogen levels in women experiencing the postpartum blues relative to women not experiencing the blues. The one finding consistent with our prediction was that free estriol showed a significantly greater drop from the average level of the prepartum assessments to the day 1 postpartum level for women experiencing the blues relative to women not experiencing the blues. There was no evidence of any role for prolactin or progesterone in the postpartum blues. There was one significant effect for total cortisol at week 38 (lower levels in women experiencing the blues), but it was not in the predicted direction. Finally, there was no association between breast-feeding status and the blues.

Implications

As noted at the beginning of this chapter, there have been relatively few significant associations observed between demographic variables and the blues in earlier research (Kennerley & Gath, 1986). However, there were a few early studies that suggested that primiparous women were at increased risk for the blues (e.g., Yalom et al., 1968) much in the way that primiparous women are at increased risk for postpartum psychosis (Kendell, 1985). We obtained no support for the possibility that primiparous women are at increased risk for the blues. Nor was there any indication in our findings that characteristics such as lower age, education, and SES were related to risk for the blues. These findings suggest that obvious potential markers for a relative lack of preparedness for childbearing in an emotional, economic, or practical sense will be of little help in identifying women at risk for the blues.

Perhaps not surprisingly, the characteristics that were most strongly associated with risk for the blues were those that indexed depressive symptoms during pregnancy and personal and family history of depression. Much like the case that we will see for postpartum depression, there appears to be a continuity of mood disturbance in these women that manifests itself in many ways. For example, women who experienced the blues were more likely to have had a past depression, premenstrual depression, high levels of depressive symptomatology during pregnancy, and postpartum depression than women who did not experience the blues. Interestingly, women who experienced the blues were not more likely to experience an RDC-defined depression during pregnancy. These observations suggest that although the blues is not primarily characterized by depressed mood, it may share some common causal factors with depression. Earlier studies have obtained inconsistent findings. For example, Kennerley and Gath (1989b) found that women who had high levels of depressive symptomatology during pregnancy were at increased risk for the blues but that there was no association between past psychiatric history and risk for the blues.

Women who experienced the blues also evidenced poorer social adjustment during pregnancy. These problems were evident in relationships with friends and family and, to a lesser extent, in the marital relationship, particularly in the second trimester. By the third trimester, women who went on to experience the blues also were more consistently complaining about their marital relationships and their adjustment to household work. These findings were in good accord with Kennerley and Gath (1989b), one of the more recent and adequate studies of the blues.

We also investigated the potential role of negative life events as a causal factor for the blues. We included not only major life events (e.g., loss of job) but also events or experiences that were thought to have more immediate impact during the postpartum period. These events included stressors related to labor and delivery (e.g., complications, problems with baby) and early childcare-related problems (e.g., trouble establishing feeding schedule). Interestingly, with respect to negative events, it was the events that occurred during the second trimester rather than the third trimester of pregnancy that were related to the blues. Perhaps these findings reflect the delayed impact of negative events, or perhaps they were a chance finding. The earlier literature has not suggested a major role for negative life events in the postpartum blues (Kennerley & Gath, 1986).

Obstetric stressors showed no association with the blues. This finding is consistent with our earlier work relating obstetric stressors to postpartum depression (O'Hara et al., 1982; O'Hara et al., 1984). Moreover, there is little evidence in the broader literature that obstetric stressors are implicated in the blues (Kennerley & Gath, 1986, 1989b). In fact, in at least two studies, higher levels of obstetric stressors were associated with lower levels of depressive symptomatology after delivery (O'Hara et al., 1982; Paykel et al., 1980). It may be that significant obstetric stressors (e.g., caesarean section) mobilize the spouse and the other members of the woman's social network in ways that more than compensate for the stress occasioned by the difficult obstetrical event (O'Hara et al., 1982).

Hospital and childcare-related stressors showed the most consistent association with indices of the blues. These events include experiences such as "Labor and/or delivery did not go the way you had hoped" and "Baby has health problems" (see Appendix A). These events all happened in close proximity to the onset of the blues and were events that, although not major, in the sense of having long-term negative implications, had a significant impact on women's day-to-day life in the early puerperium. These types of events are similar to smaller events, which are often called daily hassles (Lazarus & Folkman, 1984; Lewinsohn, Youngren, & Grosscup, 1979), and they are often significantly associated with daily mood (O'Hara & Rehm, 1979).

Because the blues occur in such close proximity to delivery and because of the dramatic decreases in reproductive hormones and, to a lesser extent, glucocorticoid hormones, these variables have been among the most extensively investigated causal factors in postpartum blues and depressive symptomatology in the early puerperium (George & Sandler, 1988; Kennerley & Gath, 1986; O'Hara, 1991). Our major hypotheses were that the blues would be associated with lower levels of the estrogens (estradiol, free and total estriol) and progesterone and higher levels of prolactin and cortisol (O'Hara, Schlechte, Lewis, & Wright, 1991; Stein, 1980; Steiner, 1979). Estrogen and progesterone withdrawal have both been posited as causal factors in reproductive-related depressions (Steiner, 1979). Moreover, Steiner (1979) suggested that low postpartum levels of estrogen and progesterone relative to prolactin may be causally related to postpartum mood disorders.

In spite of a large sample size and accurate estimations of hormone levels, there was weak support for the hormonal hypotheses. In fact, on at least 2 postpartum days, in direct contrast to our prediction, measures of free and total estriol levels were significantly *higher* in women experiencing blues than in women not experiencing the blues. As discussed in Chapter 1, the evidence for the role of hormonal factors in the puerperium has been mixed, at best, for all of the hormonal variables examined in this study. Despite the negative findings in this area, there is still considerable enthusiasm for using progesterone and estrogen and treatments for postpartum mood disorders, some of it justified (Henderson et al., 1991) and some of it unjustified (Dalton, 1982). Several of these issues will be taken up in the next two chapters.

In sum, this study represented one of the largest prospective investigations of postpartum blues to date. Although the results from the hormonal component of the study, particularly considering the large sample size, were contrary to our expectations, the analyses of the psychosocial factors did suggest that there may be a link between the affective disorders and the blues. That is, the blues may represent a marker for risk for other affective disorders, just as it did for postpartum depression in this study. Future prospective studies of the blues may illuminate risk factors for affective disorders occurring at other times.

8 Postpartum Depression

Childbearing and nonchildbearing women were followed intensively until 9 weeks postpartum. At that time all subjects were interviewed to determine whether they had experienced a major or minor depression at any time since delivery. Levels of depressive symptomatology were determined using the BDI and the SCL-90-R depression subscale at 3, 6, and 9 weeks postpartum. Subjects were asked to respond with respect to symptoms during the previous week. The major purpose of this chapter is to describe our findings regarding factors that predicted the occurrence of depression anytime in the first 9 weeks after childbirth and levels of depressive symptomatology at 3, 6, and 9 weeks after delivery.

There were several important facets of this work. First, a large sample of women was followed. The large sample size allowed for relatively powerful statistical tests of our hypotheses. Second, the study was prospective in nature and allowed us largely to disentangle the measurement of predictor and outcome variables. Third, the study was comprehensive. We were able to evaluate the role of sociodemographic variables, personal and family psychiatric history variables, social adjustment and social support variables, life stressor variables, and hormonal variables in postpartum depression. Finally, by including a nonchildbearing comparison group, we were able to observe the extent to which similar risk factors (with the exception of the hormonal variables) operate in depression in women during periods of childbearing and nonchildbearing.

This chapter is divided into two major sections. First, the relations between several classes of predictor variables and postpartum depression and levels of postpartum depressive symptomatology at 3, 6, and 9 weeks postpartum are described. The results for each of the sets of depression risk factors will be presented first for postpartum depression diagnosis. The results for childbearing and nonchildbearing subjects will be presented separately. Next, the association between depression risk factors and level of depressive symptomatology at 3, 6, and 9 weeks postpartum will be presented for childbearing and nonchildbearing subjects. Second, the results from a series of hierarchical multiple regressions that specifically test the vulnerability–life stress model of postpartum depression are presented. The model is tested separately for childbearing and nonchildbearing women, using depression diagnosis and level of depressive symptomatology (at 9 weeks postpartum) as outcomes.

We had three major hypotheses regarding the risk for RDC-defined postpartum depression. First, we predicted that personal and family history of depression would be related to postpartum depression, as we had found in our earlier work (O'Hara et al., 1983; O'Hara et al., 1984). Second, social factors, including low levels of support from spouse, families, and friends and negative life events were also expected to increase risk for depression (O'Hara, 1986; O'Hara, 1991; O'Hara et al., 1984). Finally, we expected that lower levels of the estrogens and progesterone and higher levels of prolactin and cortisol would be associated with risk for depression after delivery (O'Hara, 1991). All of these predictions were derived from our own work and the work of other postpartum depression researchers (O'Hara, 1991; O'Hara & Zekoski, 1988). With the exception of the variables that were obtained only for the childbearing subjects (hormonal measures and measures of obstetric stressors and childcare-related stressors), we made the same predictions and tested the same hypotheses with the nonchildbearing subjects.

The major hypotheses regarding depressive symptomatology at 3, 6, and 9 weeks postpartum were essentially similar to our hypotheses regarding predictors of RDC-defined depression. However, we observed in our earlier work (O'Hara et al., 1984) that somewhat different factors were associated with RDC-defined depression and high levels of depressive symptomatology. For example, self-control attitudes and level of depressive symptomatology during the second trimester were significantly associated with level of postpartum depressive symptomatology but not RDC-defined postpartum depression. These types of discrepancies may reflect the fact that depressive symptomatology and clinical depression are two different phenomena (Lewinsohn et al., 1988). Because of these considerations, we expected that measures reflecting negative cognitions and mood would be more strongly associated with postpartum depressive symptomatology than with the diagnosis of depression. Finally, there were two reasons for using both the BDI and the SCL-90-R depression subscale as outcome measures for postpartum depressive symptomatology. The BDI was chosen because we have used it in our previous research and also because it has been used in much of the postpartum depression research conducted by other investigators, particularly in the United State. The SCL-90-R depression subscale was used because, unlike the BDI, it has very few somatic items. The relative absence of somatic items is a desirable characteristic because of the possibility that scores on measures like the BDI, which has several somatic items, may be artifactually elevated by the normal somatic changes that occur during pregnancy and in the early puerperium.

Results

Demographic Factors

Depression Diagnosis

The only demographic variable to differentiate depressed and nondepressed childbearing subjects was religion, $\chi^2(6; N = 182) = 19.98$, $p < .01$. Depressed subjects were more likely to be Protestant and less likely to be Catholic. The same pattern was observed for the depressed and nondepressed nonchildbearing subjects, $\chi^2(6; N = 177) = 14.13$, $p < .05$.

Depressive Symptomatology

With respect to depressive symptomatology in childbearing subjects, none of the demographic variables were associated with level of depressive symptomatology at the 3-, 6-, or 9-week postpartum assessments.

For the nonchildbearing subjects, there were several associations between demographic variables and postpartum depressive symptomatology. At 3 weeks postpartum, there was a significant negative association between age and BDI score ($r = -.20$, $p < .01$). At both 6 weeks, $t(57.9) = 2.89$, $p < .01$, and 9 weeks postpartum, $t(75.5) = 3.69$, $p < .001$, women who had lost their fathers to death had significantly lower scores on the SCL-90-R depression subscale. Also, at 9 weeks postpartum, women who had lost their mothers to death had significantly lower levels of depressive symptomatology on the BDI, $t(17.2) = 3.18$, $p < .01$, and the SCL-90-R depression subscale, $t(18.3) = 2.87$, $p = .01$.

Personal and Family History of Psychopathology

Depression Diagnosis

Depressed childbearing subjects were more likely to have experienced a previous major depression than nondepressed childbearing subjects and to have experienced a depression during the second trimester of pregnancy than nondepressed childbearing subjects (see Table 8.1). Depressed childbearing subjects also had a higher rate of lifetime history of alcoholism than nondepressed childbearing subjects. In addition, depressed childbearing subjects were more likely than nondepressed childbearing subjects to have met criteria for the Handley Blues, the Pitt Blues, and the VAS Blues. Finally, the depressed childbearing subjects were more likely than nondepressed childbearing subjects to have mothers who had a lifetime history of major depression (see Table 8.2).

Among the nonchildbearing subjects, only 2 variables reflecting personal and family history of psychopathology differentiated the depressed and nondepressed subjects (see Tables 8.3 and 8.4). Depressed nonchildbearing subjects had a greater lifetime history of dysthymia and were

TABLE 8.1. Personal history of psychopathology in childbearing depressed and nondepressed subjects.

Variable	Depressed (N = 19) (%)	Nondepressed (N = 163) (%)	χ^2
Past depression	84.2	31.3	20.49**
Pregnancy depression	26.3	5.5	7.64*
Postpartum blues			
Handley	63.2	22.1	14.78**
Pitt	73.7	38.0	8.89*
VAS	55.6	29.4	7.47*
Premenstrual major depression	42.1	27.0	1.90
Dysthymia	0	1.2	<1
Cyclothymia	0	1.8	<1
Hypomania	0	3.7	<1
Alcoholism	36.8	4.9	18.92**
Generalized anxiety	10.5	3.1	<1

*$p < .01$
**$p < .001$
Note: All indices except premenstrual major depression were derived from the second-trimester interview. Premenstrual major depression was derived from the Premenstrual Assessment Form (Halbreich et al., 1982).

more likely to have met the Handley Blues criteria than nondepressed nonchildbearing subjects.

DEPRESSIVE SYMPTOMATOLOGY—3 WEEKS POSTPARTUM

The following variables were related to level of depressive symptomatology among the childbearing subjects on the BDI: (1) history of previous major depression, $t(178) = 4.67, p < .001$; (2) premenstrual major depression, $t(178) = 3.09, p < .01$; (3) lifetime history of hypomania; $t(178) = 2.68, p < .01$; (4) postpartum blues (Handley criteria), $t(178) =$

TABLE 8.2. Family history of psychopathology in childbearing depressed and nondepressed subjects.

Family member	Depressed (N = 19) (%)	Nondepressed (N = 163) (%)	χ^2
Depressed sibling	36.8	20.9	1.66
Depressed mother	36.8	11.0	7.51*
Depressed father	10.5	12.3	<1
Depressed partner	10.5	12.3	<1
Partner with alcohol problem	21.0	10.4	<1

*$p < .01$
Note: All indices were derived from the second-trimester interview.

TABLE 8.3. Personal history of psychopathology in nonchildbearing depressed and nondepressed subject.

Variable	Depressed (N = 14) (%)	Nondepressed (N = 164) (%)	χ^2
Past depression	42.9	39.6	<1
Pregnancy depression	7.1	5.5	<1
Premenstrual major depression	28.6	21.3	<1
Dysthymia	21.4	2.4	7.80*
Cyclothymia	7.1	3.7	<1
Hypomania	14.3	6.1	<1
Alcoholism	21.4	6.1	2.50
Generalized anxiety	0	7.9	<1

*$p < .01$

Note: All indices except premenstrual major depression were derived from the second-trimester interview. Premenstrual major depression was derived from the Premenstrual Assessment Form (Halbreich et al., 1982).

6.27, $p < .001$; and (5) depression in a first-degree relative, $t(178) = 2.72$, $p < .01$. For the SCL-90-R depression subscale, the pattern of findings was similar. The following variables were related to SCL-90-R depression subscale scores: (1) history of previous major depression, $t(178) = 4.45$, $p < .001$; (2) depression during pregnancy, $t(178) = 4.16$, $p < .001$; (3) premenstrual major depression, $t(178) = 2.78$, $p < .01$; (4) lifetime history of hypomania, $t(178) = 2.81$, $p < .01$; (5) postpartum blues (Handley criteria), $t(51.7) = 6.72$, $p < .001$; and (6) depression in a first-degree relative, $t(178) = 3.01$, $p < .01$.

The following variables were related to level of depressive symptomatology among the nonchildbearing subjects on the BDI: (1) previous history of depression, $t(107.3) = 3.80$, $p < .001$; (2) history of premenstrual major depression, $t(173) = 4.60$, $p < .001$; (3) lifetime history of alcoholism, $t(173) = 4.48$, $p < .001$; and (4) postpartum blues (Handley criteria), $t(11.6) = 3.47$, $p < .01$. The following variables were related to

TABLE 8.4. Family history of psychopathology in nonchildbearing depressed and nondepressed subjects.

Family member	Depressed (N = 14) (%)	Nondepressed (N = 164) (%)	χ^2
Depressed sibling	21.4	21.3	<1
Depressed mother	35.7	16.5	2.07
Depressed father	14.3	10.4	<1
Depressed partner	21.4	9.8	<1
Partner with alcohol problem	21.4	8.5	1.21

Note: All indices were derived from the second-trimester interview.

SCL-90-R depression subscale scores: (1) history of previous major depression, $t(91.1) = 3.43$, $p < .01$; (2) depression during pregnancy, $t(173) = 2.67$, $p < .01$; (3) premenstrual major depression, $t(173) = 3.36$, $p < .01$; and (4) postpartum blues (VAS criteria), $t(31.2) = 4.08$, $p < .001$.

Depressive Symptomatology—6 Weeks Postpartum

For the childbearing subjects, history of premenstrual major depression, $t(174) = 3.08$, $p < .01$, and postpartum blues, $t(174) = 5.68$, $p < .001$, were related to level of depressive symptomatology on the BDI. For the SCL-90-R depression subscale measure of depression, the pattern of findings was similar; however, several additional variables were predictive of the SCL-90-R scores. The following variables were related to SCL-90-R depression subscale scores: (1) history of previous major depression, $t(174) = 3.12$, $p < .01$; (2) depression during pregnancy, $t(174) = 4.00$, $p < .001$; (3) premenstrual major depression, $t(174) = 3.43$, $p < .01$; (4) lifetime history of alcoholism, $t(174) = 2.99$, $p < .01$; (5) postpartum blues (Handley criteria), $t(56.7) = 4.89$, $p < .001$, and; (6) depression in a first-degree relative, $t(174) = 2.81$, $p < .01$.

For the nonchildbearing subjects, only history of premenstrual major depression, $t(41.7) = 3.79$, $p < .001$, was related to level of depressive symptomatology on the BDI. History of premenstrual major depression, $t(42.2) = 3.38$, $p < .001$, history of dysthymia, $t(168) = 2.84$, $p < .01$, and depression during pregnancy, $t(168) = 3.44$, $p < .01$, were all related to level of depressive symptomatology on the SCL-90-R depression subscale.

Depressive Symptomatology—9 Weeks Postpartum

The following variables were related to level of depressive symptomatology among the childbearing subjects on the BDI: (1) history of previous major depression, $t(178) = 4.33$, $p < .001$; (2) depression during pregnancy, $t(178) = 3.21$, $p < .01$; (3) premenstrual major depression, $t(178) = 3.36$, $p < .01$; and (4) postpartum blues (Handley criteria), $t(178) = 5.69$, $p < .001$. For the SCL-90-R depression subscale, the following variables were related to level of depressive symptomatology: (1) history of previous major depression, $t(177) = 4.35$, $p < .001$; (2) depression during pregnancy, $t(177) = 4.73$, $p < .001$; (3) premenstrual major depression, $t(177) = 4.50$, $p < .001$; (4) postpartum blues (Handley criteria), $t(177) = 7.59$, $p < .001$; and (5) depression in a first degree relative, $t(177) = 2.62$, $p = .01$.

For nonchildbearing subjects, only history of premenstrual major depression was related to level of depressive symptomatology on the BDI, $t(44.6) = 3.73$, $p < .01$. For the SCL-90-R depression subscale, history of premenstrual major depression, $t(44.0) = 3.48$, $p < .01$, and postpartum blues (Handley criteria), $t(11.5) = 3.52$, $p < .01$, were related to level of depressive symptomatology.

Social Support During Pregnancy and After Delivery

Depression Diagnosis

There were no differences between depressed and nondepressed childbearing women with respect to social support during pregnancy and after delivery from the women's confidants, parents, and partners. The same pattern was observed for the depressed and nondepressed nonchildbearing women.

Depressive Symptomatology—3 Weeks Postpartum

For the childbearing subjects, the only social support variable that was significantly correlated with level of depressive symptomatology on the BDI was social support from the partner after delivery, $r = .21$, $p < .01$. For the SCL-90-R depression subscale, subjects' general satisfaction with support during pregnancy, $r = .21$, $p < .01$, and support from partners after delivery, $r = .22$, $p < .01$, were related to level of depressive symptomatology.

For the nonchildbearing subjects, the following social support variables were related to level of depressive symptomatology on the BDI: partner support during pregnancy, $r = .22$, $p < .01$, and partner support after delivery, $r = .23$, $p < .01$. There were no significant associations between the SCL-90-R depression subscale and measures of social support.

Depressive Symptomatology—6 Weeks Postpartum

For the childbearing subjects, the following social support variables were related to level of depressive symptomatology on the BDI: general satisfaction with support during pregnancy, $r = .24$, $p < .01$, and support from partners after delivery, $r = .22$, $p < .01$. For the SCL-90-R depression subscale, both general satisfaction with support during pregnancy, $r = .34$, $p < .001$, partner support after delivery, $r = .25$, $p < .01$, and general satisfaction with support after delivery, $r = .23$, $p < .01$, were associated with level of depressive symptomatology.

For the nonchildbearing subjects, the following social support variables were related to level of depressive symptomatology on the BDI: (1) partner support during pregnancy, $r = .25$, $p < .01$; (2) general satisfaction with support during pregnancy, $r = .23$, $p < .01$; and (3) partner support after delivery, $r = .31$, $p < .001$. For the SCL-90-R depression subscale, partner support during pregnancy, $r = .31$, $p < .001$, and partner support after delivery, $r = .26$, $p < .01$, were associated with level of depressive symptomatology.

Depressive Symptomatology—9 Weeks Postpartum

For the childbearing subjects, the following social support variables were related to level of depressive symptomatology on the BDI: (1) general satisfaction with support during pregnancy, $r = .32$, $p < .001$; (2) partner support after delivery, $r = .24$, $p < .01$; and (3) frequency that partners help with childcare, $r = .20$, $p = .01$. For the SCL-90-R depression subscale, the following variables were related to level of depressive symptomatology: (1) partner support during pregnancy, $r = .26$, $p < .01$; (2) expectation during pregnancy that spouse will help with childcare after delivery, $r = .23$, $p < .01$; (3) general satisfaction with support during pregnancy, $r = .37$, $p < .001$; (4) partner support after delivery, $r = .29$, $p < .01$; (5) frequency that partners help with childcare, $r = .28$, $p < .001$; and (6) general satisfaction with support after delivery, $r = .26$, $p < .001$.

For the nonchildbearing subjects, the following social support variables were related to level of depressive symptomatology on the BDI: general satisfaction with support during pregnancy, $r = .19$, $p = .01$, and partner support after delivery, $r = .22$, $p < .01$. There were no significant associations between the SCL-90-R depression subscale and social support variables.

Discrepancy Between Desired and Received Social Support

Depression Diagnosis

Childbearing subjects completed the Postpartum Social Support Questionnaire at 6 weeks postpartum. Discrepancies between the amount of support received and desired were assessed for partners, parents, in-laws, other relatives, and friends. On the Postpartum Social Support Questionnaire, the depressed childbearing subjects relative to nondepressed childbearing subjects reported a greater discrepancy between the actual and the desired amount of social support that they received from relatives, $t(173) = 2.30$, $p < .05$. See Table 8.5.

Depressive Symptomatology—6 Weeks Postpartum

Among the childbearing subjects the following variables were related to level of depressive symptomatology on the BDI: (1) support discrepancy for relatives, $r = .20$, $p < .01$; and (2) support discrepancy for friends, $r = .27$, $p < .001$. For the SCL-90-R depression subscale, the following variables were related to level of depressive symptomatology: (1) support discrepancy for partners, $r = .30$, $p < .001$; (2) support discrepancy for parents, $r = .21$, $p < .01$; (3) support discrepancy for relatives, $r = .25$, $p < .01$; and (4) support discrepancy for friends, $r = .31$, $p < .001$.

TABLE 8.5. Means and standard deviations of discrepancies between actual and desired levels of postpartum support by depressed and nondepressed childlbearing subjects from the Postpartum Social Support Questionnarie.

	Group	
Source of support	Depressed	Nondepressed
Partner		
M	1.39	.96
SD	.81	.57
Parents		
M	1.27	.99
SD	.90	.83
Parents-in-law		
M	1.32	.87
SD	1.09	.92
Other relatives		
M	1.48	.97
SD	1.08	.87
Friends		
M	1.07	.79
SD	.79	.77

Note: Higher scores represent greater discrepancies between actual and desired levels of support.

DEPRESSIVE SYMPTOMATOLOGY—9 WEEKS POSTPARTUM

Among the childbearing subjects, the following variables were related to level of depressive symptomatology on the BDI: (1) support discrepancy for partners, $r = .31, p < .001$; (2) support discrepancy for parents, $r = .20, p < .01$; (3) support discrepancy for relatives, $r = .23, p < .01$; and (4) support discrepancy for friends, $r = .32, p < .001$. For the SCL-90-R depression subscale, the following variables were related to level of depressive symptomatology: (1) support discrepancy for partners, $r = .37, p < .001$; (2) support discrepancy for relatives, $r = .24, p < .01$; and (3) support discrepancy for friends, $r = .39, p < .001$.

Negative Life Events

DEPRESSION DIAGNOSIS

Depressed childbearing subjects experienced a greater number of negative life events during pregnancy and after delivery than the nondepressed childbearing subjects, $t(180) = 2.02, p < .05$ (see Table 8.6). There were no significant differences between depressed and nondepressed subjects with respect to the number of negative life events during each of the trimesters of pregnancy or the 9 weeks after delivery, nor were there any differences between depressed and nondepressed childbearing subjects with respect to number of childcare-related stressors after delivery or the number of stressful events specifically related to pregnancy, labor, and delivery (see Table 8.7). Among the nonchildbearing subjects, only number of negative life events occurring after delivery differentiated the depressed and nondepressed subjects, $t(176) = 2.75$, $p < .01$.

TABLE 8.6. Means and standard deviations of number of negative life events during pregnancy and after delivery among depressed and nondepressed childbearing and nonchildbearing subjects.

Group	Depressed	Nondepressed
	First trimester	
Childbearing		
M	.84	.82
SD	1.12	1.23
Nonchildbearing		
M	.71	.72
SD	.61	1.02
	Second trimester	
Childbearing		
M	.95	.57
SD	1.18	1.00
Nonchildbearing		
M	.93	.43
SD	1.49	.77
	Third trimester	
Childbearing		
M	.63	.48
SD	1.01	1.01
Nonchildbearing		
M	.36	.44
SD	.84	.89
	After delivery	
Childbearing		
M	1.74	.86
SD	2.38	1.21
Nonchildbearing		
M	1.36	.57
SD	1.39	1.00
	Pregnancy and postpartum period combined	
Childbearing		
M	4.16	2.74
SD	2.65	2.91
Nonchildbearing		
M	3.36	2.16
SD	2.50	2.35

Table 8.7. Means and standard deviations for Peripartum Events Scale and the Childcare Stress Inventory among depressed and nondepressed childbearing subjects.

Scale	Group	
	Depressed	Nondepressed
Peripartum Events Scale		
M	5.42	5.42
SD	1.92	2.94
Childcare Stress Inventory		
M	8.37	5.91
SD	5.77	3.85

Depressive Symptomatology—3 Weeks Postpartum

Among the childbearing subjects, the following variables were related to level of depressive symptomatology on the BDI: (1) number of childcare-related-stressors, $r = .51$, $p < .001$; and (2) number of negative events in the third trimester, $r = .23$, $p < .01$. For the SCL-90-R depression subscale, only the number of childcare-related stressors was related to level of depressive symptomatology, $r = .51$, $p < .001$. None of the life event variables was related to level of depressive symptomatology among the nonchildbearing women.

Depressive Symptomatology—6 Weeks Postpartum

Among the childbearing subjects, the following variables were related to level of depressive symptomatology on the BDI: (1) number of childcare-related stressors, $r = .51$, $p < .001$; (2) number of negative events in the first trimester, $r = .21$, $p < .01$; and (3) number of negative events in the third trimester, $r = .26$, $p < .001$. For the SCL-90-R depression subscale, the following variables were related to level of depressive symptomatology: (1) number of childcare-related stressors, $r = .51$, $p < .001$; (2) number of negative events in the first trimester, $r = .19$, $p < .01$; (3) number of negative events in the second trimester, $r = .19$, $p < .01$; and (4) number of negative events in the third trimester, $r = .23$, $p < .01$. Among nonchildbearing subjects the following variables were related to level of depressive symptomatology on the BDI: (1) number of negative events in the first trimester, $r = .18$, $p < .01$; and (2) number of negative events after delivery, $r = .33$, $p < .001$.

Depressive Symptomatology—9 Weeks Postpartum

Among the childbearing subjects, the following variables were related to level of depressive symptomatology on the BDI: (1) number of childcare-related stressors, $r = .32$, $p < .001$; (2) number of negative events in the second trimester, $r = .25$, $p < .001$; (3) number of negative events in the third trimester, $r = .27$, $p < .001$; and (4) number of negative events after delivery, $r = .30$, $p < .001$. For the SCL-90-R depression subscale, the following variables were related to level of depressive symptomatology: (1) number of childcare-related stressors, $r = .35$, $p < .001$; (2) number of negative events in the second trimester, $r = .21$, $p < .01$; (3) number of negative events in third trimester, $r = .18$, $p < .01$; and (4) number of negative events after delivery, $r = .24$, $p < .01$. For the nonchildbearing subjects, both the BDI, $r = .29$, $p < .001$, and the SCL-90-R depression subscale, $r = .27$, $p < .001$, were related to number of negative events after delivery. The BDI was also related to number of negative events in the first trimester, $r = .19$, $p < .01$.

Social Adjustment During Pregnancy and After Delivery

Depression Diagnosis

In the third trimester, depressed childbearing subjects reported poorer overall adjustment than nondepressed childbearing subjects, $t(177) = 2.26$, $p < .05$ (see Table 8.8). At 3 weeks postpartum, depressed childbearing subjects relative to nondepressed childbearing subjects reported poorer overall adjustment, $t(179) = 4.19$, $p < .001$, poorer adjustment in housework-related activities, $t(179) = 2.29$, $p < .05$, poorer adjustment in relationships with extended family, $t(179) = 3.59$, $p < .001$, and poor adjustment in relationships with friends, $t(179) = 3.83$, $p < .001$. At 6 weeks postpartum, depressed childbearing subjects relative to nondepressed childbearing subjects reported poorer overall adjustment, $t(175) = 2.96$, $p < .01$, and poorer relationships with friends, $t(175) = 2.43$, $p < .05$. At 9 weeks postpartum, depressed childbearing subjects relative to nondepressed childbearing subjects reported poorer overall adjustment, $t(178) = 4.70$, $p < .001$, poorer marital adjustment, $t(25.2) = 3.63$, $p < .01$, poorer relationships with extended families, $t(178) = 2.34$, $p < .05$, and poorer relationships with friends, $t(178) = 3.97$, $p < .001$. Depressed childbearing subjects also reported significantly poorer marital adjustment on the Dyadic Adjustment Scale than nondepressed childbearing subjects at 9 weeks postpartum, $t(168) = -2.41$, $p < .05$. At 6 months postpartum, depressed childbearing subjects reported poorer overall adjustment, $t(160) = 2.71$, $p < .01$, poorer marital adjustment, $t(146) = 2.84$, $p < .01$, and poorer adjustment in relations with extended families, $t(160) = 2.72$, $p < .01$.

During the second trimester, depressed nonchildbearing subjects relative to nondepressed nonchildbearing subjects reported poorer overall social adjustment, $t(176) = 3.42$, $p < .01$, poorer relationships with extended families, $t(175) = 2.07$, $p < .05$, poorer relationships with friends, $t(176) = 2.98$, $p < .01$, and poorer adjustment in work at home,

TABLE 8.8. Means and standard deviations of social and marital adjustment scales among depressed and nondepressed childbearing and nonchildbearing subjects during the second trimester of pregnancy through 6 months postpartum.

	Group			
	Childbearing		Nonchildbearing	
Scale	Depressed	Nondepressed	Depressed	Nondepressed
	Second trimester			
SAS-SR				
Marital relationship	2.09	1.89	1.93	1.81
	(.41)	(.40)	(.37)	(.41)
Family relationships	1.70	1.54	1.74	1.55
	(.37)	(.37)	(.41)	(.33)
Relationships with friends	2.19	2.02	2.16	1.85
	(.65)	(.52)	(.49)	(.36)
Work at home	1.96	1.93	2.27	1.89
	(.44)	(.50)	(.43)	(.42)
Overall adjustment	1.94	1.82	1.97	1.74
	(.28)	(.34)	(.34)	(.24)
Dyadic Adjustment Scale	106.37	113.24	99.82	111.53
	(20.43)	(15.10)	(25.88)	(15.20)
	Third trimester			
SAS-SR				
Marital relationship	2.20	1.98	1.79	1.77
	(.59)	(.48)	(.44)	(.46)
Family relationships	1.63	1.50	1.71	1.54
	(.42)	(.34)	(.43)	(.36)
Relationships with friends	2.04	1.93	2.23	1.86
	(.55)	(.45)	(.62)	(.42)
Work at home	2.08	1.86	2.07	1.83
	(.53)	(.50)	(.64)	(.46)
Overall adjustment	1.97	1.78	1.91	1.71
	(.41)	(.32)	(.42)	(.30)
	3 weeks postpartum			
SAS-SR				
Marital relationship	2.38	2.22	1.77	1.77
	(.61)	(.45)	(.44)	(.47)
Family relationships	1.85	1.54	1.55	1.51
	(.40)	(.35)	(.28)	(.45)
Relationships with friends	2.36	1.92	2.22	1.82
	(.51)	(.47)	(.72)	(.42)
Work at home	2.12	1.84	2.14	1.79
	(.61)	(.51)	(.62)	(.48)
Overall adjustment	2.21	1.88	1.92	1.68
	(.45)	(.31)	(.46)	(.32)
	6 weeks postpartum			
SAS-SR				
Marital relationship	2.18	2.03	1.91	1.74
	(.47)	(.49)	(.47)	(.45)
Family relationships	1.62	1.45	1.62	1.44
	(.44)	(.35)	(.45)	(.38)

TABLE 8.8. *Continued*

Scale	Group			
	Childbearing		Nonchildbearing	
	Depressed	Nondepressed	Depressed	Nondepressed
Relationships with friends	2.07	1.83	2.29	1.80
	(.36)	(.42)	(.86)	(.44)
Work at home	1.92	1.74	2.19	1.76
	(.39)	(.48)	(.64)	(.51)
Overall adjustment	1.98	1.75	1.92	1.64
	(.29)	(.30)	(.53)	(.32)
		Second trimester		
SAS-SR				
Marital relationship	2.17	1.85	1.72	1.70
	(.32)	(.49)	(.38)	(.42)
Family relationships	1.63	1.44	1.68	1.40
	(.37)	(.34)	(.55)	(.33)
Relationships with friends	2.28	1.86	2.27	1.76
	(.52)	(.42)	(.61)	(.43)
Work at home	1.88	1.70	2.33	1.75
	(.30)	(.47)	(.73)	(.50)
Overall adjustment	1.99	1.68	1.94	1.61
	(.28)	(.27)	(.48)	(.31)
Dyadic Adjustment Scale	102.79	113.62	105.45	113.47
	(24.07)	(17.66)	(17.67)	(15.18)
		6 months postpartum		
SAS-SR				
Marital relationship	2.34	1.88	1.78	1.74
	(.65)	(.54)	(.36)	(.50)
Family relationships	1.70	1.45	1.72	1.45
	(.38)	(.34)	(.86)	(.40)
Relationships with friends	2.19	1.95	2.16	1.80
	(.56)	(.51)	(.52)	(.41)
Work at home	1.87	1.69	2.06	1.70
	(.35)	(.48)	(.59)	(.45)
Overall adjustment	1.96	1.70	1.87	1.62
	(.37)	(.34)	(.43)	(.31)

$t(176) = 3.21$, $p < .01$ (see Table 8.8). During the third trimester, depressed nonchildbearing subjects relative to nondepressed nonchildbearing subjects reported poorer overall social adjustment, $t(173) = 2.35$, $p < .05$, and poorer adjustment with friends, $t(14.0) = 2.21$, $p < .05$. At 3 weeks postpartum, depressed nonchildbearing subjects relative to nondepressed nonchildbearing subjects reported poorer adjustment in work at home, $t(171) = 2.45$, $p < .05$. At 6 weeks postpartum, depressed nonchildbearing subjects relative to nondepressed nonchildbearing subjects reported poorer adjustment in work at home, $t(169) = 2.89$, $p <$

.01. At 9 weeks postpartum, depressed nonchildbearing subjects relative to nondepressed nonchildbearing subjects reported poorer overall social adjustment, $t(175) = 3.74$, $p < .001$, poorer relationships with friends, $t(14.5) = 3.10$, $p < .01$, and poorer adjustment to work at home, $t(174) = 4.02$, $p < .001$. At 6 months postpartum, depressed nonchildbearing subjects evidenced poorer overall adjustment, $t(152) = 2.71$, $p < .01$, poorer adjustment with friends, $t(152) = 2.92$, $p < .01$, and poorer adjustment in work at home, $t(152) = 2.70$, $p < .01$.

Depressive Symptomatology

Among the childbearing subjects, based on the SAS-SR, overall level of social adjustment, adjustment in work at home, marital adjustment, adjustment in relationships with extended families, and adjustment in relationships with friends assessed in the second and third trimesters and at 3, 6, and 9 weeks postpartum were, almost without exception, significantly associated with levels of depressive symptomatology measured by the BDI and the SCL-90-R depression subscale at 3, 6, and 9 weeks postpartum (see Table 8.9). Similar findings were obtained for the nonchildbearing subjects (see Table 8.9).

Table 8.9. Association between social adjustment and levels of depressive symptomatology among childbearing and nonchildbearing subjects during the third, sixth, and ninth week postpartum.

Social Adjustment Scale subscales	Group: Childbearing BDI	Childbearing SCL-90-R	Nonchildbearing BDI	Nonchildbearing SCL-90-R
	Week 3 postpartum			
Marital relationship	.43	.49	.50	.48
Family relationships	.47	.48	.52	.52
Relationships with friends	.42	.51	.57	.51
Work at home	.56	.61	.49	.41
Overall adjustment	.66	.73	.74	.71
	Week 6 postpartum			
Marital relationship	.38	.45	.47	.51
Family relationships	.45	.40	.56	.63
Relationships with friends	.54	.53	.64	.63
Work at home	.54	.56	.48	.50
Overall adjustment	.68	.71	.75	.76
	Week 9 postpartum			
Marital relationship	.37	.41	.49	.44
Family relationships	.36	.33	.57	.58
Relationships with friends	.47	.45	.54	.56
Work at home	.41	.46	.47	.51
Overall adjustment	.64	.66	.75	.76

Note: All correlations are significant, at least $p < .001$.

Subjects also completed the Dyadic Adjustment Scale in the second trimester and at 9 weeks postpartum. For the childbearing subjects, marital adjustment in the second trimester measured by the DAS was significantly related to level of depressive symptomatology measured by the BDI at 6 weeks postpartum, $r = -.22$, $p < .01$, and the SCL-90-R depression subscale $r = -.21$, $p < .01$. Second-trimester DAS score was also related to the level of depressive symptomatology at 9 weeks postpartum on the SCL-90-R depression subscale, $r = -.22$. The DAS obtained at 9 weeks postpartum was related to level of depressive symptomatology assessed at 9 weeks postpartum for both the BDI, $r = -.28$, $p < .001$, and the SCL-90-R depression subscale, $r = -.31$, $p < .001$.

Similar findings were obtained for the nonchildbearing subjects. Second-trimester DAS score was significantly related to level of depressive symptomatology at (1) 3 weeks postpartum on the BDI, $r = -.24$, $p < .01$; (2) 6 weeks postpartum on the BDI, $r = -.30$, $p < .001$, and the SCL-90-R depression subscale, $r = -.28$, $p < .001$; and (3) 9 weeks postpartum on the BDI, $r = -.29$, $p < .01$, and the SCL-90-R depression subscale, $r = -.27$, $p < .01$. The DAS obtained at 9 weeks postpartum was related to level of depressive symptomatology assessed at 9 weeks postpartum for both the BDI, $r = -.35$, $p < .001$, and the SCL-90-R depression subscale, $r = -.32$, $p < .001$.

Self-Control Attitudes

Depression Diagnosis

Self-control attitudes were assessed with the Self-Control Questionnaire in the second trimester and at 9 weeks postpartum. For childbearing subjects there were no differences between childbearing depressed and nondepressed subjects for SCQ assessed during pregnancy or after delivery. The nonchildbearing depressed subjects had significantly more dysfunctional self-control attitudes after delivery than the nondepressed subjects, $t(174) = 2.00$, $p < .05$. However, the prenatal difference between nonchildbearing depressed and nondepressed subjects was not significant.

Depressive Symptomatology

For the childbearing subjects, self-control attitudes in the second trimester measured by the SCQ were significantly related to level of depressive symptomatology at 6 weeks postpartum measured by the BDI, $r = .25$, $p < .001$, and the SCL-90-R depression subscale, $r = .24$, $p < .01$. Second-trimester SCQ score was also related to the level of depressive symptomatology at 9 weeks postpartum as measured by the BDI, $r = .23$, $p < .01$, and the SCL-90-R depression subscale, $r = .21$, $p < .01$. The SCQ obtained at 9 weeks postpartum was related to level of depressive symptomatology assessed at 9 weeks postpartum on the BDI, $r = .20$, $p < .01$.

For the nonchildbearing subjects, self-control attitudes in the second trimester measured by the SCQ were significantly related to level of depressive symptomatology at 6 weeks postpartum measured by the BDI, $r = .21, p < .01$. The SCQ obtained at 9 weeks postpartum was related to level of depressive symptomatology assessed at 9 weeks postpartum on the BDI, $r = .23$, $p < .01$, and the SCL-90-R depression subscale, $r = .28$, $p < .001$.

Biological Factors

Hormonal data were available for 18 of the 19 childbearing women who had experienced a postpartum depression. There were a few occasions, particularly week 38 of gestation and day 1 postpartum, when 1 or 2 (and on 2 occasions, 3) depressed women missed their blood draw. Multivariate analyses of variance were conducted for each of the reproductive and glucocorticoid hormones comparing postpartum-depressed and -nondepressed women. There were no significant effects for group (depressed vs. nondepressed) or for the interaction term (Group X Assessment Occasion) for any of the hormonal variables. However, there were several significant differences between depressed and nondepressed subjects for estradiol and total cortisol on individual days; they are described in the next two sections.

Reproductive Hormones

Depressed subjects had significantly lower levels of estradiol at week 36 of gestation, $t(36.0) = 2.79$, $p < .01$, and at day 2 postpartum, $t(50.1) = 3.06$, $p < .01$, (see Table 8.10). There were no differences between depressed and nondepressed subjects for free estriol and total estriol for any of the assessment occasions. Moreover, there were no significant differences between depressed and nondepressed subjects for progesterone and prolactin for any of the assessment occasions. Finally, there were no significant differences between depressed and nondepressed subjects for the ratios of prolactin to estradiol or progesterone for any of the assessment occasions.

Glucocorticoid Hormones

Depressed subjects had significantly lower levels of total cortisol at week 38 of gestation, $t(152) = 2.40$, $p < .05$, and at day 2 postpartum, $t(168) = 2.25$, $p < .05$. There were no other differences between depressed and nondepressed subjects for total plasma cortisol or for urinary free cortisol at any of the assessments (see Table 8.11). With respect to dexamethasone suppression, nonsuppression was defined as a 7:00 A.M. or 4:00 P.M. post dexamethasone cortisol $>5\,\mu g/dl$. There was a very high rate of nonsuppression at both the 7:00 A.M. assessment (92.1%) and the 4:00 P.M.

assessment (93.8%). The differences between depressed and nondepressed subjects were not significant at either assessment.

Tests of a Vulnerability–Life Stress Model of Postpartum Depressive Symptomatology

Five sets of variables were entered into the hierarchical multiple regression: (1) sociodemographic, (2) depression history vulnerability, (3) social and cognitive vulnerability, (4) life stress, and (5) vulnerability–life stress interactions. The sociodemographic set included (a) age, (b) working status during pregnancy, (c) marital status, and (d) socioeconomic status (Hollingshead, 1975). The sociodemographic set was not of theoretical interest in our model; rather, the variables in that set were included as control variables. The second set reflected vulnerability to depression based on depression history. Its variables included (a) number of previous episodes of depression, (b) whether a first-degree family member had ever been depressed, (c) whether the subject had a major or minor depression during pregnancy, and (d) the second-trimester BDI score. The third set reflected social and cognitive vulnerability to depression and were (a) marital adjustment (the DAS) and (b) self-control attitudes (the SCQ). The life stress set included (a) the number of negative life events since the beginning of pregnancy (the PLES), (b) the number of stressful life events associated with late pregnancy, labor, and delivery (peripartum events—the PES), and (c) the number of childcare-related stressors since delivery (the CSI). The latter 2 measures were excluded in the regressions involving the nonchildbearing women. The vulnerability–life stress interactions were entered last. There were 18 interaction terms (3 life stress measures × 6 vulnerability measures) for childbearing subjects and 6 interaction terms (1 life stress measure × 6 vulnerability measures) for nonchildbearing subjects. The 9-week postpartum BDI score was the measure of postpartum depressive symptomatology.

Childbearing Subjects

The overall F from the multiple regression was highly significant (see Table 8.12). The depression history vulnerability, life stress, and vulnerability–life stress sets of predictor variables were significant in the regression. Similar to our earlier studies (O'Hara et al., 1982; O'Hara et al., 1984), depression level during pregnancy showed the strongest association with postpartum depressive symptomatology. In contrast to our more recent study (O'Hara et al., 1984), number of previous depressions was significant in the multiple regression. The depression history vulnerability set accounted for 19% of the variance in postpartum depressive symptomatology. The number of stressful life

TABLE 8.10. Prepartum and postpartum levels of reproductive hormones for childbearing postpartum-depressed and -nondepressed subjects.

	Week of gestation			Postpartum day					
Hormone	34	36	38	1	2	3	4 (A.M.)	6	8
Estradiol (pmol/d)									
Depressed									
M	27,367	25,344	28,411	2,952	1,226	588	504	355	265
SD	12,420	9,969	12,692	1,788	582	318	315	185	127
Nondepressed									
M	30,034	33,296	35,741	3,852	1,786	732	526	387	315
SD	15,886	19,539	20,302	3,005	1,484	461	321	259	171
Total estriol (nmol/d)									
Depressed									
M	311	375	510	116	70	32	18	2.9	1.2
SD	123	161	234	56	64	28	23	4.3	1.9
Nondepressed									
M	359	459	623	122	73	34	14	3.0	1.7
SD	165	254	343	87	68	35	23	5.2	3.8
Free estriol (nmol/d)									
Depressed									
M	44	51	66	5.5	2.9	2.1	1.8	.7	.5
SD	28	36	31	5.2	2.5	2.1	2.0	.9	.6
Nondepressed									
M	44	54	73	4.5	3.1	2.0	1.2	.6	.4
SD	20	25	35	5.1	3.7	2.6	1.5	.9	.6

Progesterone (nmol/L)									
Depressed									
M	309	306	421	52	19	8.5	6.7	2.9	2.0
SD	177	178	289	68	19	9.7	5.6	2.0	1.2
Nondepressed									
M	309	369	407	46	17	9.0	6.8	3.0	2.2
SD	198	273	278	42	10	5.8	4.1	2.0	1.9
Prolactin (μg/L)									
Depressed									
M	176	228	212	192	186	202	178	154	113
SD	90	181	151	130	82	144	135	121	75
Nondepressed									
M	178	190	208	168	219	169	178	137	136
SD	77	77	84	96	119	77	98	86	141

Note: Sample sizes ranged from 148 to 169; smaller sample sizes usually occurred at week 38 of gestation because some subjects had delivered. From "Controlled prospective study of postpartum mood disorders: Psychological, environmental, and hormonal variables" by M.W. O'Hara, J.A. Schlechte, D.A. Lewis, & M.W. Varner, 1991, *Journal of Abnormal Psychology, 100,* 63–73. Copyright 1991 by the American Psychological Association. Adapted by permission of the publisher.

TABLE 8.11. Prepartum and postpartum levels of glucocorticoid hormones for childbearing postpartum-depressed and -nondepressed subjects.

	Week of gestation			Postpartum day						
Hormone	34	36	38	1	2	3	4 (A.M.)	4 (P.M.)	6	8
Total cortisol (nmol/L)										
Depressed										
M	922	879	773	780	583	641	357	458	711	689
SD	277	342	242	360	219	250	292	159	308	263
Nondepressed										
M	908	920	920	758	726	696	332	414	733	690
SD	255	242	238	255	260	225	215	214	214	224
Urinary free cortisol (nmol/d)										
Depressed										
M	220	236	253		228		116			
SD	81	76	70		134		66			
Nondepressed										
M	232	228	230		195		118			
SD	99	92	85		125		101			

Note: Sample sizes ranged from 152 to 173; smaller sample sizes usually occurred at week 38 of gestation because some subjects had delivered. From "Controlled prospective study of postpartum mood disorders: Psychological, environmental, and hormonal variables" by M.W. O'Hara, J.A. Schlechte, D.A. Lewis, & M.W. Varner, 1991, *Journal of Abnormal Psychology, 100,* 63–73. Copyright 1991 by the American Psychological Association. Adapted by permission of the publisher.

TABLE 8.12. Hierarchical multiple regression of postpartum depression level (based on BDI) on demographic, vulnerability, and life stress factors for childbearing subjects[a].

Predictor variable	r	R	ΔR^2	R^2	Standardized β	F	df	$t(136)$
Sociodemographic		.209	.044	.044		1.86	4,136	
Socioeconomic status	−.152				−.175			
Working during pregnancy	.077				.056			
Marital status	−.105				−.074			
Age	.033				.145			
Depression history vulnerability		.487	.193	.237		10.08***	4,136	
No. of previous episodes of depression	.299***				.209			2.84**
Depressed first-degree relative	−.128				−.055			<1
Depressed during pregnancy	−.213**				.020			<1
Second-trimester Beck Depression Inventory	.435***				.367			4.44***
Social and cognitive vulnerability		.500	.013	.250		1.38	2,136	
Self-Control Questionnaire	.256**				.124			
Dyadic Adjustment Scale	−.201**				−.028			
Life stress		.575	.081	.331		6.20***	3,136	
Pilkonis Life Events Scale	.370***				.216			2.67**
Peripartum Events Scale	.117				.056			<1
Childcare Stress Inventory	.304***				.171			2.25*
Vulnerability–life stress[b]		.708	.171	.502		2.59**	18,136	

*$p < .05$
**$p < .01$
***$p < .001$
[a] $F(31, 136) = 4.42, p < .001$
[b] See text for the specific interaction terms that were significant in the regression
Note: The tests for the zero order correlations are one-tailed. From "Controlled prospective study of postpartum mood disorders: Psychological, environmental, and hormonal variables" by M.W. O'Hara, J.A. Schlechte, D.A. Lewis, & M.W. Varner, 1991, *Journal of Abnormal Psychology, 100,* 63–73. Copyright 1991 by the American Psychological Association. Reprinted by permission of the publisher.

TABLE 8.13. Hierarchical multiple regression of postpartum depression level (based on BDI) on demographic, vulnerability, and life stress factors for nonchildbearing subjects[a].

Predictor variable	r	R	ΔR^2	R^2	Standardized β	F	df	$t(147)$
Sociodemographic		.295	.087	.087		3.81**	4,147	
Socioeconomic status	−.172				−.116			<1
Working during pregnancy	.163				.136			1.76
Marital status	−.248**				−.194			−2.14*
Age	−.117				.030			<1
Depression history vulnerability		.659	.347	.434		23.93***	4,147	
No. of previous episodes of depression	.226**				.099			1.54
Depressed first-degree relative	−.078				−.055			<1
Depressed during pregnancy	−.104				−.045			<1
Second-trimester Beck Depression Inventory	.627***				.591			9.15***
Social and cognitive vulnerability		.660	.002	.436		<1	2,147	
Self-Control Questionnaire	.107				−.039			
Dyadic Adjustment Scale	−.281***				−.034			
Life stress		.687	.036	.472		10.48**	1,147	
Pilkonis Life Events Scale	.338***				.209			
Vulnerability–life stress		.710	.032	.504		1.57	6,147	

*$p < .05$
**$p < .01$
***$p < .001$
[a] $F(17, 147) = 8.79, p < .001$
Note: The tests for the zero order correlations are one-tailed. From "Controlled prospective study of postpartum mood disorders: Psychological, environmental, and hormonal variables" by M.W. O'Hara, J.A. Schlechte, D.A. Lewis, & M.W. Varner, 1991, *Journal of Abnormal Psychology, 100*, 63–73. Copyright 1991 by the American Psychological Association. Reprinted by permission of the publisher.

events since delivery and the number of childcare-related stressors were also significant in the multiple regression. As a group, the life stress set accounted for 8% of the variance in postpartum depressive symptomatology. The set of vulnerability–life stress interactions was also highly significant accounting for an additional 17% of the variance. Within that group the following interactions were significant ($p < .05$): "self-control attitudes by negative life events" [$t(136) = -3.11$], "prepartum depression by childcare-related stressors" [$t(136) = 2.97$], and "prepartum depression by peripartum life events" [$t(136) = -2.33$].

Nonchildbearing Subjects

The overall F from the multiple regression for the nonchildbearing subjects was also highly significant (see Table 8.13). The sociodemographic, depression history vulnerability, and life stress sets were significant. For nonchildbearing subjects being married at the time of the second-trimester interview was significantly associated with lower levels of postpartum depressive symptomatology. Within the depression history vulnerability set, the prepartum BDI was the only significant variable; and it, along with the other variables in this set, accounted for 35% of the variance in postpartum depressive symptomatology. Finally, number of negative life events was a significant predictor of postpartum depressive symptomatology, accounting for 4% of the variance.

Tests of a Vulnerability–Life Stress Model of Postpartum Depression Diagnosis

Childbearing Women

The same variables were entered in the same order in the multiple regression of postpartum depression diagnostic status as for the multiple regression of postpartum depressive symptomatology. Once again, the overall F was highly significant (see Table 8.14). The pattern of results showed some similarities to the earlier regression. Two sets of variables were significant: depression history vulnerability and vulnerability–life stress. Within the depression history vulnerability set, which accounted for 16% of the variance in postpartum depression diagnosis, number of previous depressions and depression during pregnancy were the significant predictors. The vulnerability–life stress set accounted for another 19% of the variance. Within that set there were two significant interaction terms ($p < .05$): "number of previous depressions by number of childcare-related stressors" [$t(136) = -3.61$] and "prepartum depression by peripartum events" [$t(136) = 4.64$].

TABLE 8.14. Hierarchical multiple regression of postpartum depression diagnostic status on demographic, vulnerability, and life stress factors for childbearing subjects.[a]

Predictor variable	r	R	ΔR^2	R^2	Standardized β	F	df	$t(136)$
Sociodemographic		.201	.040	.040		1.72	4,136	
Socioeconomic status	−.136				−.168			
Working during pregnancy	.000				−.021			
Marital status	−.123				−.097			
Age	.041				.140			
Depression history vulnerability		.452	.164	.204		8.18**	4,136	
No. of previous episodes of depression	.371***				.348			4.64**
Depressed first-degree relative	−.150				−.097			−1.31
Depressed during pregnancy	.248**				.163			−2.01*
Second-Trimester Beck Depression Inventory	.179**				−.028			<1
Social and cognitive vulnerability		.452	.001	.205		<1	2,136	
Self-Control Questionnaire	.112				.007			
Dyadic Adjustment Scale	−.150				−.026			
Life stress		.462	.009	.213		<1	1,136	
Pilkonis Life Events Scale	.149				−.042			
Peripartum Events Scale	.000				−.010			
Childcare Stress Inventory	.174**				.106			
Vulnerability–life stress[b]		.635	.190	.404		2.41**	18,136	

*$p < .05$
**$p < .01$
***$p < .001$
[a] $F(31, 136) = 2.97$, $p < .001$
[b] See Results section for the specific interaction terms that were significant in the regression
Note: The tests for the zero order correlations are one-tailed. From "Controlled prospective study of postpartum mood disorders: Psychological, environmental, and hormonal variables" by M.W. O'Hara, J.A. Schlechte, D.A. Lewis, & M.W. Varner, 1991, *Journal of Abnormal Psychology, 100,* 63–73.

NONCHILDBEARING WOMEN

The overall F from the multiple regression for nonchildbearing subjects was also significant (see Table 8.15). Only the vulnerability–life stress set was significant, and within that set only the "BDI during pregnancy by negative life events" interaction was significant [$t(147) = -2.06, p < .05$].

Summary

Depression Diagnosis

Personal and family history of depression were the major risk factors for postpartum depression for childbearing subjects. History of depression before and during pregnancy, premenstrual major depression, postpartum blues, and having a mother with a history of depression were all associated with depression in the postpartum period. In a related vein, postpartum-depressed childbearing subjects showed evidence of poor social adjustment beginning in the second trimester of pregnancy and extending through 9 weeks postpartum. Negative life events, through pregnancy and the postpartum period, were elevated for depressed childbearing subjects; however, postpartum-depressed subjects did not show elevated levels of either childcare-related stressors early in the puerperium or stressors associated with labor and delivery. Also, there was little evidence of any differences between depressed and nondepressed subjects with respect to social support from parents, confidants, and partners during pregnancy or the puerperium. Finally, the hormonal variables yielded differences between depressed and nondepressed subjects in levels of estradiol only on 2 occasions.

The variables in the vulnerability–life stress model accounted for about 40% of the variance in postpartum depression diagnosis in childbearing subjects. Two vulnerability variables, number of previous episodes of depression and depression during pregnancy, were significant predictors of postpartum depression. In addition, two of the interaction terms were also significant.

The overall pattern of findings with respect to predictors of depression for nonchildbearing subjects was similar to the pattern of findings observed for the childbearing subjects. Depressed nonchildbearing subjects had greater lifetime histories of dysthymia and were more likely to meet criteria for the blues than nondepressed nonchildbearing subjects. Similar to the case for the childbearing subjects, depressed nonchildbearing subjects showed relatively poorer social adjustment than nondepressed nonchildbearing subjects beginning in the second trimester and continuing through the postpartum period. Depressed nonchildbearing subjects also showed higher levels of negative life events during the postpartum period than nondepressed nonchildbearing subjects.

TABLE 8.15. Hierarchical multiple regression of postpartum depression diagnostic status on demographic, vulnerability, and life stress factors for nonchildbearing subjects[a].

Predictor variables	r	R	ΔR^2	R^2	Standardized β	F	df
Sociodemographic		.046	.002	.002			4,147
Socioeconomic status	−.039				−.030	<1	
Working during pregnancy	.015				.014		
Marital status	−.033				−.014		
Age	−.029				−.009		
Depression history vulnerability		.234	.053	.055		2.17	4,147
No. of previous episodes of depression	.070				.028		
Depressed first-degree relative	−.030				−.027		
Depressed during pregnancy	.034				−.017		
Second-trimester Beck Depression Inventory	.229*				.233		
Social and cognitive vulnerability		.265	.015	.070		1.26	2,147
Self-Control Questionnaire	.101				.057		
Dyadic Adjustment Scale	−.190**				−.117		
Life stress		.287	.013	.083		2.11	1,147
Pilkonis Life Events Scale	.153				.124		
Vulnerability–life stress[b]		.419	.093	.176		2.77*	6,147

*$p < .05$
**$p < .01$
[a] $F(17, 147) = 1.84, p < .05$
[b] See Results section for the specific interaction terms that were significant in the regression
Note: The tests for the zero order correlations are one-tailed. From "Controlled prospective study of postpartum mood disorders: Psychological, environmental, and hormonal variables" by M.W. O'Hara, J.A. Schlechte, D.A. Lewis, & M.W. Varner, 1991, *Journal of Abnormal Psychology, 100,* 63–73. Copyright 1991 by the American Psychological Association. Reprinted by permission of the publisher.

The vulnerability–life stress model accounted for only about 18% of the variance in depression diagnosis among the nonchildbearing subjects. However, there were fewer predictor variables (the PES and the CSI were not appropriate for the nonchildbearing subjects). Only the group of interaction variables (BDI during pregnancy X negative life events) was significant in the regression.

Depressive Symptomatology

A wide variety of the depression history variables was related to depressive symptomatology at 3, 6, and 9 weeks postpartum. Similarly, almost all indices of social adjustment showed a significant association with measures of depressive symptomatology after delivery. With respect to social support, general satisfaction with support during pregnancy and support from the women's partners were the social support variables that showed the most consistent association with postpartum depressive symptomatology. There was also a consistent association between discrepancy between actual and desired support from social network members and level of depressive symptomatology. In addition, several indices of negative life events were significantly associated with level of postpartum depressive symptomatology. However, Peripartum Events Scale scores were not associated with level of depressive symptomatology at any time in the postpartum period. Finally, dysfunctional self-control attitudes measured during the second trimester and at 9 weeks postpartum were associated with indices of postpartum depressive symptomatology.

The vulnerability–life stress model accounted for 50% of the variance in level of depressive symptomatology at 9 weeks postpartum. The depression history vulnerability variables, the life stress variables, and the variables representing the interaction of vulnerability and life stress variables were significant predictors of level of postpartum depressive symptomatology.

Similar to the case for childbearing subjects, many of the depression history and social adjustment variables were related to level of depressive symptomatology at 3, 6, and 9 weeks postpartum. Surprisingly, having mothers or fathers who had died was significantly associated with *lower* levels of depressive symptomatology at 9 weeks postpartum. Once again, general satisfaction with support during pregnancy and support from the women's partners were the social support variables most consistently associated with level of postpartum depressive symptomatology. Unlike the case for the childbearing subjects, there was only 1 instance in which there was a significant association between number of negative life events and level of depressive symptomatology (i.e., number of negative life events after delivery and level of depressive symptomatology at 9 weeks postpartum). Also, dysfunctional self-control attitudes measured during the second trimester and at 9 weeks postpartum were associated with indices of postpartum depressive symptomatology.

In the context of the regression analysis, the second-trimester BDI was highly correlated with the 9-week postpartum BDI ($r = .63$). As a consequence, only 1 other variable, number of negative life events, was a significant predictor of level of postpartum depressive symptomatology.

Implications

One way of conceptualizing the broad array of variables that we investigated with respect to postpartum depression was in terms of vulnerability factors, stress factors, and the interaction of vulnerability and stress factors. The vulnerability–life stress model incorporated most of these factors. The major factors left out of the model were the hormonal variables. These variables were not included because we were less confident of their causal importance and because of their sheer number and the difficulty of constructing a composite index reflecting hormonal vulnerability. In this section discussion will be organized around the major elements of our model. In the next chapter, I will try to draw out the broader implications of the findings reported in this and earlier chapters.

The vulnerability–stress model of postpartum depression accounted for a significant amount of variance in depression diagnosis and in level of depressive symptomatology for both childbearing and nonchildbearing women. The major variables that emerged in each of these regressions were those that reflected "depression history vulnerability" and the interaction of the vulnerability factors (depression history and social and cognitive factors) and the stress variables. However, in almost all cases, the vulnerability factors that interacted (at a significant level) with a stress variable were those that reflected "depression history" (e.g., depression during pregnancy). These findings point to the importance of past psychopathology in accounting for the occurrence of postpartum depression. This finding replicates our earlier work and the work of others in studies of depression after childbirth (O'Hara et al., 1983; Watson et al., 1984) and depression that occurs at other times and in other contexts (Lewinsohn et al., 1988). In the next chapter, some of the practical implications of these findings for health and mental health care providers are discussed.

One of the assumptions underlying this research was that childbearing is a stressful life event (or a series of stressful life events) that should increase a woman's risk for depression. We expected that the stress of pregnancy, delivery, and early childcare would interact with many of the depression vulnerability factors discussed earlier in this chapter to increase the risk for depression relative to nonchildbearing periods. Our assumption was not supported by the data. Although childbearing women experienced higher levels of diagnosed depression during pregnancy and after delivery than nonchildbearing women, the differences were not significant. Other stressful life events, both the more general and serious ones (e.g., job loss, change of housing) and the ones specifically related to childbearing (i.e., obstetric stressors, childcare-related stressors) were evaluated directly and in interaction with depression vulnerability factors. Direct effects of life stressors were observed only in the prediction of level of postpartum depressive symptomatology; however, interaction effects were observed for both diagnosis of postpartum depression and level of depressive symptomatology.

Our diathesis–stress model of postpartum depression was supported with the childbearing group. The diatheses (or vulnerability factors) were the most potent predictive factors for postpartum depression. However, the set of "interaction of stress and vulnerability" factors accounted for about the same amount of variance as the set of "depression history vulnerability" factors in both postpartum depression diagnosis and level of depressive symptomatology. These findings suggest that even if the postpartum period, per se, is not a stressor that increases the risk for depression after childbirth, consideration of additional sources of stress, both associated and not associated with childbearing, is important in risk for postpartum depression (O'Hara, Schlechte, Lewis, & Varner, 1991).

There was little evidence in this study of a hormonal influence on risk for postpartum depression. These findings echoed the results we obtained regarding hormonal influences on the blues. With a few exceptions, neither absolute levels of the hormones nor their degree of change from late pregnancy to the early puerperium were related to diagnosis of postpartum depression. In the cases of progesterone and the estrogens, there was between a 5-fold and a 10-fold drop in levels from week 38 of gestation to day 1 postpartum. By day 8 postpartum, these changes had reached 100-fold or more for progesterone and the estrogens. Despite these rather dramatic changes, on only 2 occasions were there any significant differences between depressed and nondepressed subjects on hormonal variables—estradiol levels at week 36 of gestation and on day 2 postpartum were significantly lower for postpartum-depressed women.

As suggested in chapters 1 and 7, the literature with respect to the impact of sudden and dramatic decreases in levels of progesterone and the estrogens on postpartum mood has been quite mixed. For example, several investigators claimed that supplemental progesterone after childbirth was effective in reducing the probability of a postpartum mood disturbance (Bower & Altschule, 1956; Dalton, 1980; Solthau & Taylor,

1982). However, these studies were not controlled, and a number of other correlational studies have not found any evidence of an association between postpartum progesterone levels and postpartum mood disorders (Ballinger et al., 1982; Kuevi et al., 1983; Metz et al., 1983). The one exception to these negative findings for progesterone was a recent study (Harris et al., 1989) in which lower levels of progesterone were found in depressed breast-feeding women at about 8 weeks postpartum.

Although we found that postpartum-depressed women had lower levels of estradiol than nondepressed women on day 2 postpartum in accordance with the estrogen withdrawal hypothesis, these differences were also apparent during pregnancy and a significant effect was observed at week 36 gestation. As suggested in chapter 1, the results of earlier studies of the relation between estrogen levels and postpartum depression have been inconclusive. The major importance of our findings with respect to progesterone and the estrogens is that in spite of a large sample size, predicted associations with postpartum depression were not observed.

High levels of prolactin in nonchildbearing women are associated with depression, anxiety, and hostility (Campbell & Winokur, 1985). In chapter 1 it was indicated that the literature was mixed with respect to the association between prolactin levels and postpartum mood disturbance. For example, George et al. (1980) found, as predicted, that higher levels of prolactin were positively correlated with dysphoric mood on several postpartum days; however, in a more recent study, Harris et al. (1989) found that lower levels of prolactin were associated with level of depression at 8 weeks postpartum. Other studies, including the current one, have found no evident relation between prolactin levels and postpartum mood (e.g., Nott et al., 1976). Inconclusive findings with respect to prolactin could be due to methodological problems. For example, breast-feeding stimulates prolactin secretion, and prolactin levels are higher in breast-feeding than in non-breast-feeding women. We asked women to abstain from breast-feeding for 2 hours before blood draws; and although blood draws were done early in the morning, it is possible that artifacts associated with breast-feeding obscured differences that may have existed between depressed and nondepressed women.

There were no differences between depressed and nondepressed women with respect to either total cortisol or urinary free cortisol levels. Moreover, the rates of nonsuppression and cortisol levels following the dexamethasone suppression test were similar for depressed and nondepressed women. These findings are relatively consistent with other studies that have failed to find an association between higher levels of cortisol and postpartum mood disturbance (Handley et al., 1977; Handley et al., 1980; Kuevi et al., 1983). One recent study did find the predicted association between higher levels of salivary cortisol and postpartum blues (Ehlert et al., 1990). However, in total there is little evidence that cortisol dynamics distinguish postpartum-depressed and -nondepressed women.

The final chapter will expand on many of the themes that have been developed in this and previous chapters. There will also be a discussion of future research directions for the study of postpartum depression. Finally, the chapter will take up some issues related to the care of childbearing women by health care and mental health professionals.

9
Summary and Implications

Summary of Results

Depression During Pregnancy and After Delivery

A large percentage of both childbearing and nonchildbearing women had experienced a major depression (36% to 40%) at some point prior to their entry into our study. Rates of other psychiatric disorders were substantially lower, yet in the aggregate, these results suggest that psychological suffering was very common in the lives of the women in our study despite the fact that they averaged only about 27 years of age.

Although childbearing women had about a one-third higher rate of depression during pregnancy and after delivery than nonchildbearing women, the differences were not significant. In contrast, the postpartum blues were much more common in the childbearing than in the nonchildbearing women. Moreover, the childbearing women reported significantly higher levels of depressive symptomatology during late pregnancy and the early puerperium. These differences were reflected in the self-reports obtained from the Beck Depression Inventory and the depression subscale of the SCL-90-R as well as interview-based ratings of cognitive symptomatology. Finally, the picture revealed by the Visual Analogue Scales ratings in late pregnancy and the first week postpartum suggested that childbearing women were significantly more distressed than nonchildbearing women at the end of their pregnancies and at the end of the first postpartum week.

Social Adjustment, Support, and Stressors During Pregnancy and After Delivery

Childbearing women showed poorer social adjustment than nonchildbearing women early in the postpartum period, particularly with respect to their marital relationship. Both childbearing and nonchildbearing women reported decreases in social support from their confidants, parents, and partners over the course of the study. Childbearing women appeared to experience less support from their confidants and partners than did nonchildbearing women after delivery. Overall, childbearing women were disappointed in the amount of support that they received from all sources after their babies were born. Surprisingly, childbearing women also experienced higher levels of negative life events after delivery than the nonchildbearing women.

Predictors of Depression During Pregnancy

There were several important features that distinguished RDC-defined depressed and nondepressed childbearing women during pregnancy. With respect to sociodemographic variables, depressed women had a lower socioeconomic status. They also had a higher rate of past major depression and were more likely to have history of alcoholism than nondepressed childbearing women. Depressed women also reported lower levels of social support from their partners and more negative life events during pregnancy than nondepressed childbearing women. Finally, depressed childbearing women evidenced poorer social adjustment and more dysfunctional self-control beliefs than nondepressed women.

Depressed and nondepressed nonchildbearing women showed a pattern similar to the depressed and nondepressed childbearing women, with a few exceptions. Among sociodemographic variables only religion was related to diagnosis of depression during pregnancy. Catholics and Protestants were less likely to be depressed. Depressed nonchildbearing women were also more likely to have experienced a previous major depression and to have reported a history of premenstrual major depression and dysthymia, as well as having a partner with a lifetime history of alcoholism. Interestingly, depressed nonchildbearing women reported receiving *more* support from their confidants than nondepressed women. The depressed women also experienced more negative life events during pregnancy. Finally, depressed nonchildbearing women reported poorer social adjustment and more dysfunctional self-control beliefs during pregnancy.

Variables reflecting lower social status (e.g., lower SES, education, unemployment, being single) were associated with higher levels of depressive symptomatology during the second and third trimesters of pregnancy for both childbearing and nonchildbearing women. Again, for both childbearing and nonchildbearing women, previous psychiatric history (depression, cyclothymia, alcoholism) was associated with higher levels of depressive symptomatology during the second and third trimesters of pregnancy. For the childbearing women only, a lifetime history of alcoholism in the partner was associated with higher levels of depressive symptomatology. Lower levels of support from the partner were associated with higher levels of depressive symptomatology for both the childbearing and nonchildbearing women. In addition, parental support was important for the childbearing women. Further, for both childbearing and nonchildbearing women, higher levels of negative events in the second trimester were associated with higher levels of depressive symptomatology in the second trimester. Finally, higher levels of depressive symptomatology in the second and third trimesters were associated with poorer social adjustment and more dysfunctional self-control beliefs in both childbearing and nonchildbearing women.

Predictors of the Postpartum Blues

Childbearing women who had higher levels of depressive symptomatology and lower levels of social adjustment were at increased risk for the blues. Although past history of depression was related to increased risk for the blues, major or minor depression during pregnancy did not increase risk. With respect to social factors, women who had higher levels of negative events during the second trimester of pregnancy and who experienced higher levels of childcare-related stressors were at increased risk for the blues. In addition, women who during pregnancy expected less help with childcare from their parents and partners after delivery were at increased risk for the blues. Finally, hormonal variables were not strongly associated with the blues. However, consistent with the estrogen hypothesis, higher levels of free and total estriol during late pregnancy and greater change in levels of free estriol from pregnancy to day 1 postpartum were associated with increased risk for the blues.

Predictors of Postpartum Depression

Personal and family history of depression were the major risk factors for postpartum depression for childbearing women. Postpartum-depressed childbearing women also showed evidence of poor social adjustment during pregnancy, which continued throughout the puerperium. They also experienced higher levels of negative life events. Interestingly, there was little evidence of lower levels of social support from partners, parents, or confidants of these women. With respect to hormonal variables, lower levels of estradiol were observed late in pregnancy and early in the puerperium among the depressed women. The vulnerability–life stress model, which incorporated the demographic, depression history, social-cognitive, and life stress factors, accounted for 40% of the variance in postpartum depression. Individually, number of prior episodes of depression and depression during pregnancy along with 2 of the vulnerability by life stress interaction terms were significant predictors in the hierarchical multiple regression that tested the model.

For the nonchildbearing women, a pattern similar to that of the childbearing women emerged. Dysthymia and the blues were the depression history variables that were associated with postpartum depression. Depressed nonchildbearing women also showed higher levels of negative life events and poorer social adjustment beginning during pregnancy. The vulnerability–life stress model accounted for 18% of the variance in postpartum depression. Only 1 interaction term, BDI during pregnancy by negative life events, was a significant predictor.

A wide array of predictor variables was associated with levels of depressive symptomatology during the postpartum period. Interestingly, none of the demographic variables was associated with level of depressive symptomatology after delivery for the childbearing women. For nonchildbearing women only a few demographic variables were associated with level of depressive symptomatology (e.g., lower age with higher depression level). Many of the variables reflecting personal or family history of depression were associated with level of depressive symptomatology at the 3 postpartum assessments for both childbearing and nonchildbearing women. Social support variables were more highly associated with level of depression symptomatology after delivery than they were with postpartum depression diagnosis, for both the childbearing and nonchildbearing women. Moreover, discrepancies between actual and desired levels of support from family and friends were associated with levels of depressive symptomatology for the childbearing women. For both childbearing and nonchildbearing women, poorer social adjustment and more dysfunctional self-control beliefs beginning during pregnancy were associated with higher levels of postpartum depressive symptomatology. Finally, the vulnerability–life stress model was highly significant in predicting level of depressive symptomatology for both the childbearing and nonchildbearing women.

Implications

This study addressed several major issues that bear on the health and welfare of childbearing women. The principal foci were the relative rates of depression in childbearing and nonchildbearing women and psychological, biological, and environmental etiologic factors in postpartum depression. However, we also addressed issues of depression during pregnancy. Relatively less attention has been paid to this problem. In addition, we obtained measures of adjustment and social stress that allowed us to investigate the overall adjustment of women through the last half of pregnancy and the first 3 months postpartum. The availability of an acquaintance control group allowed us to investigate social role domains in which women are relatively disadvantaged during pregnancy and the early puerperium. The rest of this chapter will be devoted to discussing the implications of our findings in each of these areas. Additionally, the implications of the findings of this work will be addressed for the future study of the psychological consequences of childbearing.

What Is Postpartum Depression?

The rates of major and minor depression after delivery for childbearing women were not significantly higher than the rates for nonchildbearing women. Moreover, levels of depressive symptomatology were significantly higher during pregnancy that after delivery for both the childbearing and nonchildbearing women. What do these findings mean for our understanding of postpartum depression and its consequences? Is postpartum depression a useful concept or should it be abandoned, given our new understandings from this and other recent studies? In this section, a discussion and integration of the findings of the current work with the larger literature will be presented.

At the time that the current study was undertaken (1984), there was very little direct evidence regarding the extent to which women were at increased risk for depression after delivery. For example, in an earlier study, we obtained a postpartum depression prevalence rate of 12% (O'Hara et al., 1984). This rate compared to a 9% rate that we obtained for a 1-month period in the second trimester of pregnancy in the same study. Although the differences between the pregnancy and the postpartum rates were not significant, we speculated at the time that the postpartum rate of 12% was about twice what we would have expected for comparable sample of women from the community (O'Hara et al., 1984). Several important British studies were also published about this time (1982 to 1984) and came to somewhat different conclusions regarding risk for depression in the postpartum period (Cox et al., 1982; Kumar & Robson, 1984; Watson et al., 1984). In each of these studies, substantially more women were depressed in the first 6 to 12 weeks after delivery than a relatively comparable interval during pregnancy. However, Watson et al. pointed to high rates of depression observed among women in community studies. In contrast, Kumar and Robson and Cox et al. emphasized the high degree of psychiatric morbidity observed in their samples after delivery. Some of the postpartum depression cases observed in these studies began in pregnancy; however, the vast majority of cases developed after delivery, a phenomenon that we had observed as well (O'Hara et al., 1984). At this point (1984) it still seemed plausible that risk for depression increased after delivery; however, doubts were appearing regarding the extent to which that increased risk was really significant (Watson et al., 1984).

Cooper et al. (1988) addressed many of the issues that we addressed in our study. They were concerned about the relative rates of nonpsychotic psychiatric disorder (which included depressive and anxiety disorders) in childbearing and nonchildbearing women and followed a large sample of women (N = 483) from Cambridge, England, from late pregnancy through 1 year postpartum. Psychiatric status in all women was assessed at the antenatal interview; however, only a subsample of women were interviewed after delivery. For example, at 3 months postpartum, a random sample of 106 women were interviewed as well as all women who, on the basis of the General Health Questionnaire (GHQ), were probable "cases" (of psychiatric disorder) (Goldberg, 1972), and a subsample of women who, on the basis of the GHQ, were not probable cases, for a total sample of 243 women. The comparison sample of 576 nonchildbearing women had been assembled in Edinburgh, Scotland (Surtees et al., 1983). These women were selected to be similar to the childbearing women on demographic variables. Cooper et al. found little difference in rates of depressive and anxiety disorders in childbearing and nonchildbearing subjects at 3 and 6 months postpartum. Moreover, there were relatively few significant differences in the nature of psychiatric disorders across the childbearing and nonchildbearing subjects. The results were largely in agreement with the observations of Watson et al. (1984) regarding rates of depression observed in community studies. Nevertheless, the comparison subjects in the Cooper et al. study were drawn from a different city and "country" than the childbearing subjects and were assessed on only one occasion rather than the multiple occasions for the childbearing subjects. Finally, only subsamples of the childbearing subjects were interviewed during the puerperium, raising the possibility that some postpartum depressions were missed. Our study did not have these limitations yet came to many of the same conclusions.

Troutman and Cutrona (1990) used procedures very similar to those in the current study and followed childbearing and nonchildbearing (acquaintance controls) adolescents from the second trimester of pregnancy until 1 year postpartum. These 128 childbearing and 114 nonchildbearing adolescents ranged in age from 14 to 18 years. This study, the only postpartum depression study of adolescents, found high rates of RDC-defined major and minor depression at each assessment, ranging from 16% during pregnancy to 26% (6% major, 20% minor) at 6 weeks postpartum. Interestingly, the rates for the nonchildbearing adolescents were also high, 17% during pregnancy and 15% at 6 weeks postpartum. These rates were not significantly different, despite the apparent large difference at 6 weeks postpartum. Troutman and Cutrona's findings point to the ubiquitousness of depression in young women and the importance of an appropriate control group in interpreting the significance of such high rates of depression in adolescent mothers.

The results of a recent study (Cox et al., 1993) raise the intriguing possibility that childbirth may affect the timing of the onset of depression if not actually increase the risk of depression. In a study of 232 childbearing women and an equal number of matched controls, Cox et al. used a two-stage screening process (similar to Cooper et al., 1988) and determined that the point prevalence at 6 months postpartum and the 6-month period prevalence rates of depression were similar in both groups. However, three times as many childbearing subjects as control subjects had episodes of depression that began in the first 5 weeks after childbirth. Also, many of the depressed control subjects had episodes of long-standing duration, some following a previous childbirth. The issue of timing of postpartum episodes will be discussed shortly.

The results of the current study and other recent studies (Cooper et al., 1988; Cox et al., 1993; Troutman & Cutrona, 1990) suggest that a woman's risk for nonpsychotic depression is not increased after childbirth. The qualifier "nonpsychotic" is used because of the convincing evidence that risk for psychotic episodes (including depression, mania, schizophrenia, and other functional psychoses) does increase substantially in the first 30 to 60 days after delivery (Kendell et al., 1987). However, in Kendell et al.'s (1987) classic epidemiological study of 54,087 births, of the 120 women who were hospitalized during pregnancy or within 3 months of delivery, 47% were not psychotic and, in fact, 17% were suffering from only a minor depression. Nevertheless, the relative risk of being hospitalized for a psychotic episode in the first 30 days after delivery was 21.7, whereas the relative risk of being hospitalized for any psychiatric disorder (psychotic or not) was 6.0. These findings suggest that a woman's risk for hospitalization for psychiatric disorder is increased (as much as 6-fold in the puerperium) and a woman's risk for hospitalization for a psychotic disorder is very greatly increased (as much as 21-fold) in the early puerperium. In summary, it is most accurate to say that only a woman's risk for a *nonpsychotic* depression *not requiring hospitalization* is not increased during the puerperium.

Although the prevalence of depression may not be increased during the puerperium, there is some evidence that depressions tend to occur in relatively close proximity to childbirth. For example, Kumar and Robson (1984) observed 16 new cases of depression at 3 months postpartum but only 5 new cases each at 6 months and 1 year postpartum. Watson et al. (1984) found that 67% of depression episodes beginning in the first year postpartum occurred within 3 months of delivery. Cooper et al. (1988) reported that 40% of new episodes began in the first 3 months postpartum. In Cox et al. (1993), 50% of postpartum depressed childbearing women had episodes that began within 5 weeks of delivery. The comparable percentage for their control sample was 16%, which was significantly less. However, Nott (1987) did not observe this pattern. Finally, we found that for 69% of our postpartum-depressed subjects, their episodes of depression began within 3 weeks of delivery. Nevertheless, an equal percentage of nonchildbearing depressed subjects had an episode that began within 3 weeks postpartum as well. These findings suggest that depressions that begin in the months following childbirth may occur earlier rather than later in the puerperium. However, our findings also suggest the *possibility* that depression after childbirth may be particularly salient to a woman. Some subjects may be expecting that a depression should occur after delivery or are otherwise ready to report on symptoms occurring after childbirth when asked. Another possibility is that using childbirth as an anchor in an interview to determine the onset of symptoms may cause some women to identify their symptoms as beginning early in the puerperium, for example, rather than late in pregnancy. Only a phenomenon of this sort would explain the fact that so many of our depressed nonchildbearing subjects reported that their depressions began within the first few weeks postpartum.

Depressions that occur after childbirth may show a symptom pattern different from depressions that occur other times. For example, Pitt (1968) argued in his seminal study that depressions occurring after childbirth are "atypical." "Atypical" depression was meant to characterize those depressions that had prominent neurotic symptoms, such as anxiety, irritability, or phobias, which tended to overshadow the depression. Pitt suggested that many of the women experiencing a postpartum depression in his sample had these "atypical" depression characteristics (see also Nieland & Roger, 1993). Similar arguments have been made for the distinctiveness of postpartum psychosis (Brockington et al., 1981; Dean & Kendell, 1981). However, Cooper et al. (1988) found no support for this view in comparing the symptom pictures of depressed childbearing and nonchildbearing women. Moreover, we saw little evidence of differences in symptom pictures, with the exception that at 3 weeks postpartum the depressed childbearing subjects had significantly higher levels of depressive symptomatology than the depressed nonchildbearing subjects. Whiffen and Gotlib (1993) found few differences between samples of depressed childbearing and nonchildbearing women. Women experiencing postpartum depression tended to have less severe episodes and better marital relationships than depressed nonchildbearing women. Unfortunately, in the only other controlled study (Troutman & Cutrona, 1990), there was no report on possible symptom differences that may have characterized their depressed childbearing and nonchildbearing adolescents. Although there has been little indication of distinct symptoms that characterize depressed childbearing women (Purdy & Frank, 1993), too little research has addressed this question for us to be confident that postpartum depression does not present in some distinctive fashion.

Given that there is little evidence that depression after childbirth occurs at a rate higher than at other times in a woman's life, and given that there is only modest evidence that depressions may cluster around delivery or have particularly distinct features, is there any reason to continue to specifically target for attention depressions that occur in the puerperium? The answer is yes, and there are a number of reasons, many of which were reviewed in chapter 1. However, the major reason is that depressions occurring in the postpartum period may reflect an ongoing vulnerability to affective disorder. Our finding of a heavy loading of past depression in women who experience postpartum depressions (O'Hara, Schlechte, Lewis, & Varner, 1991) and the results of several follow-up studies indicating that women who experience postpartum depression continue to be vulnerable to depression in the years following childbirth (Ghodsian et al., 1984; Kumar & Robson, 1984; Philipps & O'Hara, 1991) suggest that postpartum depression may be a good marker of ongoing risk for depression. Given that most depressions go unidentified and untreated by mental health professionals (Shapiro et al., 1984), and given that childbearing women are in regular contact with health care professionals, the postpartum period may be the ideal time to identify and treat depressed women without engaging in costly community screening programs (Philipps & O'Hara, 1991). Moreover, there is now a rather substantial literature suggesting that parental depression (mothers or fathers) is associated with a host of behavioral and emotional problems in children of all ages (Downey & Coyne, 1990; Gelfand & Teti, 1990). In fact, recent research suggests that children of depressed mothers may be specifically vulnerable to depression (Hammen, 1991). Identifying and treating depressed childbearing women would have the advantages of reducing unnecessary suffering in women, reducing a major stressor for most families (i.e., the stress of having a depressed mother/wife), and decreasing the likelihood that the child will be exposed to a depressed mother over a long period of time.

Causes of Postpartum Depression

In this study there were two depression outcomes, clinical diagnosis, reflected in the Research Diagnostic Criteria for major and minor depression, and level of depressive symptomatology, reflected in the scores on the Beck Depression Inventory and the SCL-90-R. Defining depression in terms of a syndrome through the use of diagnostic criteria has the advantage of being relatively objective and designating a minimal (1) constellation of symptoms, (2) symptom severity, and (3) duration of episode. Diagnostic criteria also serve to rule out alternative explanations for observed symptoms (e.g., another psychiatric or medical disorder). The recent major studies of postpartum depression have defined depression in this way and, in some cases, in other ways as well (Cooper et al., 1988; Gotlib et al., 1991; Troutman & Cutrona, 1990; Whiffen, 1988). The other major way to define depression is in terms of level of depressive symptomatology based on a self-report or interview-based measures such as we used in this study (Troutman & Cutrona, 1990; Whifen, 1988).

Although many studies of postpartum depression, including this one, have used scores on depression inventories as measures of postpartum depression level, the question of whether these kinds of measures actually quantify amount of postpartum depression in the absence of a prior determination of the presence of the postpartum depression (e.g., through a diagnostic interview) is open to debate. Lewinsohn, Hoberman, and

Rosenbaum (1988) have argued that the BDI and other similar instruments measure nonspecific negative affect (Watson & Tellegen, 1985), high levels of which way be necessary but are not sufficient for a diagnosis of depression. Lewinsohn et al. point to a study by Breslau (1985) in which a self-report measure of depression detected generalized anxiety as well as depression. Also, it is common for measures of depression and other constructs such as anxiety to be highly correlated (Gotlib, 1984). For example, the correlation between our measures of depression and anxiety was $r = .73$ at 9 weeks postpartum. Moreover, it is very clear that many individuals who score at high levels on measures of depressive symptomatology are not depressed when examined clinically. This approach suggests that level of depressive symptomatology might be better thought of as an index of psychological adjustment. This perspective would reduce the confusion surrounding the inconsistencies that we and others (Lewinsohn et al., 1988) have frequently observed regarding predictors of depression defined on the basis of either diagnosis or depression severity measures. This perspective also would suggest that in future studies, measures such as the SCL-90-R (Derogatis, 1983), which taps a large number of symptom dimensions, would be superior to a relatively narrow measure like the BDI if the investigator is interested in assessing this aspect of postpartum adjustment.

Sociodemographic Variables

There was little evidence from our study that sociodemographic factors were associated with postpartum depression in childbearing or nonchildbearing women. Social disadvantage (e.g., lower SES, education, and occupation level; younger age; being single) would seem to be a plausible risk factor for postpartum depression (Brown & Harris, 1978). All of these factors should make adaptation to the demands of being a new mother more difficult. Nevertheless, there has been very little evidence in the postpartum depression literature that sociodemographic variables are consistently related to the occurrence of depression after childbirth. Other social factors may be more important during the puerperium. For example, medical anthropologists have argued that postpartum depression is much less common in non-Western countries and cultures where social stressors associated with low education and occupational status and poverty may be quite common (Harkness, 1987; Stern & Kruckman, 1983). They suggest that there are many elements of the social structuring of the postpartum period that are present in non-Western cultures but are missing in the United States and Europe. These anthropologists would argue that social advantage is not nearly as important as having postpartum rituals that support and value the new mother. Unfortunately, in the current study and in other major studies of postpartum depression, there have been no attempts to investigate the social structuring of the postpartum period in individual families and to relate this social structuring to the woman's risk for depression.

Psychopathology Variables

In most of our studies, women who have experienced episodes of depression prior to their pregnancies have been at increased risk for postpartum depression (O'Hara et al., 1983; O'Hara, Schlechte, Lewis, & Varner, 1991). Similar findings from prospective studies of postpartum depression were obtained by Watson et al. (1984) but not by Kumar and Robson (1984). Our findings are consistent with those of a large prospective community study of depression that included men and women (Lewinsohn et al., 1988) and with the literature on risk for postpartum psychosis (Kendell, 1985; O'Hara, 1991). Depression is a recurrent disorder, with an average risk of recurrence of about 50% (Belsher & Costello, 1988). As a consequence, at any given point in time, a woman who has had a previous depression is more at risk for becoming depressed than a woman who has never been depressed. This was the finding of Lewinsohn et al. (1988). If we accept that the early puerperium is a stressful time for women, we might expect that women who had previously experienced a depressive episode would be at particular risk for an episode during the puerperium.

In our study 84% of women who experienced a postpartum depression, as compared to 31% of women who did not experience a postpartum depression, had a history of depression prior to pregnancy (see Table 8.1). To put it another way, childbearing women who had experienced a depression prior to pregnancy had a 23.9% prevalence of postpartum depression, as compared to a prevalence of 2.6% for women who had not experienced a previous depression. We did not find this to be the case for the nonchildbearing women. The nonchildbearing women who experienced a postpartum depression were no more likely to have had a past history of depression than the nonchildbearing women who did not experience a postpartum depression. Moreover, nonchildbearing women who had experienced a depression prior to pregnancy did not have a higher rate of postpartum depression than nonchildbearing women who had not experienced a previous depression. These results suggest that, for our subjects, the presence of the stressful event of childbearing may have been necessary to activate the vulnerability for depression associated with having had a past depression.

In contrast to what we reported in O'Hara et al. (1984), we found that depression during pregnancy was associated with increased risk for postpartum depression. Among the postpartum-depressed women, 26% had been depressed at the time of the second-trimester interview (many of whom were the same women who had past depressions). In fact, 5 of 14 women who were depressed at the time of the second-trimester interview experienced a postpartum depression. Interestingly, the percentages of women who did and did not experience a postpartum depression and who were depressed during pregnancy were about the same in the earlier study; however, because the sample size of that study was much smaller than the current study, the differences between the postpartum-depressed and -nondepressed subjects were not significant. We had argued in an earlier paper that depressions during pregnancy may be atypical, in the sense that they reflect the presence of somatic symptoms associated with the physical discomfort of pregnancy and that they may be relieved by childbirth (O'Hara, 1986). Three of the 12 women who had experienced a postpartum depression were depressed in the second trimester. In contrast, Kumar and Robson (1984) found that all but 1 of their pregnancy depressions had remitted before delivery. Only 1 of their 17 postpartum-depressed subjects had been depressed at 36 weeks gestation (though they might have been depressed earlier in pregnancy).

The other major psychopathology predictors of postpartum depression were the postpartum blues and a past history of alcoholism. Paykel et al. (1980) also found that the blues was associated with later depression. However, there is no clear way that the blues can be distinguished from an early onset postpartum depression. Although the definitions of our various indices of the blues were not the same as the diagnostic criteria we used for depression, there was substantial overlap, particularly for the Pitt and Handley definitions. The blues measure based on the Visual Analogue Scales completed by women during the first week postpartum was probably most distinct from the diagnostic assessments of postpartum depression conducted at 9 weeks postpartum. The blues will be discussed more in a later section; however, the presence of the blues can serve to alert the clinician to the possibility that a more serious depressive disorder is in the offing. Clearly, more work is necessary to determine the natural history of the blues and whether it can be distinguished from the early stages of a postpartum depression.

Past history of alcoholism was the only significant nondepression psychopathology risk factor for postpartum depression. It was associated with depression in pregnancy as well. However, most of what was diagnosed as alcoholism in this study reflected abusive drinking at a younger age, often when women were in their late teens and early twenties. No woman admitted to abusive drinking during or immediately before pregnancy. Alcoholism has been linked to depression both theoretically and empirically (Lehman, 1985; Cadoret & Winokur, 1974). Past alcohol abuse may serve as a general marker for depression vulnerability, much like past depression. Interestingly, past history of alcoholism was not associated with increased risk for depression in the nonchildbearing subjects.

Depression does run in families (Hammen, 1991). However, the familial link in postpartum depression has not been evaluated in many studies

(O'Hara & Zekoski, 1988). There seems to be good evidence that family history of mental illness is associated with an increased risk of postpartum psychosis; however, the picture for postpartum depression is not as clear. In an earlier study (O'Hara et al., 1984), we found that depression in first-degree relatives (mother, father, siblings) was associated with increased risk for postpartum depression. Watson et al. (1984) found that family psychiatric history was associated with risk for postpartum depression, though at a marginal significance level. Kumar and Robson (1984) found that psychiatric disorder in either parent was not associated with risk for postpartum depression.

The evidence for a familial link for postpartum depression in the current study was equivocal. Overall, there was no association between depression in first-degree relatives and postpartum depression; however, women whose mothers had experienced depression at some time in their lives were at increased risk for postpartum depression. Interestingly, among the depressed nonchildbearing women, the rate of depression in subjects' mothers was equivalent to that for depressed childbearing women; however, the nondepressed nonchildbearing women had a higher rate of depression in their mothers than the nondepressed childbearing women.

The findings regarding the potential links between postpartum depression and personal and familial psychopathology suggest that psychopathology risk factors operate in much the same way for postpartum depression and depressions that occur at other times and in other contexts. In most studies in which these factors have been investigated, some element of psychopathology risk has been found to be associated with postpartum depression (O'Hara, 1991; O'Hara & Zekoski, 1988). It may be that these indices of past personal and family psychopathology are indexing some feature (biological or behavioral) that pushes a woman from simply being dysphoric and unhappy after delivery (i.e., high levels of depressive symptomatology) to developing the syndrome of depression (see Lewinsohn et al., 1988, for a similar argument).

Although we will discuss some of the practical implications of this and other recent studies for the obstetrical and psychological care of childbearing women later in this chapter, this perspective does suggest the need to carefully monitor women after childbirth who have a past personal and family history of depression. This monitoring as a prelude to early intervention is important for two reasons. First, it reflects our understanding that women with past depression are at increased risk for depression after childbirth. Second, it helps women and their families to be alert for changes in functioning that reflect the onset of a depressive episode. In sum, both our theoretical understanding of postpartum depression and our practical care of childbearing women must reflect the link between previous personal and family psychopathology and postpartum depression.

Social and Cognitive Variables

There was very little evidence from this study that social support from the partner, parent, or confidant was related to postpartum depression in either the childbearing or nonchildbearing subjects. This result was the single most anomalous finding from our study. It stands in contrast to our findings in earlier studies (O'Hara, 1986; O'Hara et al., 1983) in which we used very similar methodology with very similar subjects and found that lower levels of social support, particularly from the spouse, were significantly related to increased risk for postpartum depression. Our findings were also in contrast to findings of other studies of postpartum depression and depression occurring at other times that have suggested that social support is important in reducing risk for depression in otherwise vulnerable women (Brown & Harris, 1978; Gotlib et al., 1991; Paykel et al., 1980). Only Hopkins et al. (1987) obtained findings similar to our own. They speculated that, overall, their sample was characterized by a high level of marital satisfaction (even the depressed subjects) and that all subjects were receiving a minimum amount of social support. The women in our study were somewhat more heterogeneous than the subjects in Hopkins et al. (1987), and their overall level of marital satisfaction was considerably lower than subjects in Hopkins et al. However, we cannot explain our findings through the logic of the Hopkins et al. argument.

Two other measures that indirectly measured social support from the spouse were the marital adjustment subscale from the SAS-SR and the Dyadic Adjustment Scale. Women who experienced a postpartum depression reported lower levels of marital adjustment (from SAS-SR) during the second trimester of pregnancy and poorer marital adjustment (SAS-SR and DAS) at 9 weeks postpartum. These findings were more in accord with the literature (O'Hara & Zekoski, 1988) than the findings from our more direct measures of social support. In earlier studies we had consistently found that support from the spouse was the most important element of social support. A good marital relationship greatly increases the likelihood that the partner will provide the instrumental and emotional support necessary to reduce childcare and other burdens of his wife during the puerperium.

Stressors

The number of negative life events occurring from the beginning of pregnancy through 9 weeks postpartum was associated with increased risk for postpartum depression. Interestingly, the number of negative events occurring only after delivery was not associated with risk for postpartum depression. There also was no direct association between number of obstetrically related peripartum events or childcare-related stressors and postpartum depression. However, both of these stress variables interacted with depression vulnerability variables (presence of pregnancy depression and number of previous depressions, respectively) to account for significant variance in predicting postpartum depression. These findings suggest that the direct effects of stress and the effects of stress in the presence of depression vulnerability factors put a woman at increased risk for postpartum depression. The direct effects of stress have been documented in several of our earlier studies (O'Hara, 1986; O'Hara et al., 1983) and in other major studies (Gotlib et al., 1989; Paykel et al., 1980). Two recent studies found that infant-related stressors (e.g., medical difficulties) but not other types of stressful life events were related to increased risk for depression (Hopkins et al., 1987; Whiffen, 1988). A few studies have found no evidence to support a role for stressors in postpartum depression (Kumar & Robson, 1984; Pitt, 1968). Finally, Martin et al. (1989) have argued that psychosocial stressors may be more important determinants of depression during pregnancy than after delivery. They found, using George Brown's Bedford College Life Events and Difficulties Schedule (Brown & Harris, 1978), that 89% of the cases of depression occurring during pregnancy and only 40% of cases occurring after delivery could be attributed to the presence of a provoking agent (a severe life event). The authors suggested that psychosocial stressors played less of a role in postpartum depressions than prepartum depressions and depressions occurring at other times and that biological factors may play a more important role in postpartum depression.

There would seem to be little question that severe life events or major difficulties are related to increased risk for depression (Brown & Harris, 1989; Monroe & Simons, 1991). The work of Brown and his colleagues suggests that individual severe events are much more likely to cause a depression than an accumulation of less severe events (Brown & Harris, 1978; 1989; Martin et al., 1989). However, the results of a number of other prospective studies of postpartum and nonpostpartum depression have found that accumulating negative life events do lead to depression (Gotlib et al., 1991; Lewinsohn et al., 1988; O'Hara, 1986). Moreover, the results of our study and the work of Brown and Harris (1978; 1989) suggest that the conjunction of life stressors and vulnerability factors is especially important in accounting for risk for depression. Our vulnerability factors reflected a predisposition to depression (e.g., past depression), while Brown and Harris's (1978) vulnerability factors included a broad array of current and past social factors (no confiding relationship with partner, 3 or more children under age 14, early loss of mother, and no outside employment). Together, these studies suggest that for childbearing women who experience an especially negative event and who also have had a history of depression or a negative social situation, depression will not be an unexpected consequence. In fact, it may be that these are women who should be targeted for preventive interventions to reduce the likelihood of a postpartum depression.

Hormonal Factors

As stated early in this volume, the evidence for a hormonal etiology for postpartum depression is quite weak. The results of our study did little to alter that impression of the literature. There was little evidence that levels of progesterone, prolactin, or cortisol had any relation to risk for postpartum depression, or blues for that matter. These null findings are in general accord with the literature to date, including studies published since this study was undertaken. The most relevant exception was the finding by Harris et al. (1989) who found that lower levels of prolactin were associated with higher levels of depression. They also found that the effects of progesterone differed depending upon whether the woman was breast-feeding or bottle-feeding. Among bottle-feeders, higher levels of progesterone were associated with higher levels of depressive symptomatology. However, just the opposite association was observed for breast-feeders. These findings were not consistent with expectations regarding the effects of prolactin and progesterone but do suggest that consideration of a woman's breast-feeding status may be important in considering the effects of hormonal factors.

Only estrogen levels evidenced any association with postpartum depression or the blues in our study. The findings for estrogen levels were few, with some in the predicted direction and others not in the predicted direction. Moreover, there is little evidence from other studies that estrogen levels are related to postpartum depression or the blues. Interestingly, two studies are currently under way that involve treatment of postpartum depression using transdermal estrogen (Henderson et al., 1991) and estrogen prophylaxis for women at high risk for postpartum psychosis (Kumar, 1991). As described in chapter 1, preliminary data suggest that estrogen may be an effective treatment for postpartum depression. However, full analysis of the results of these very interesting treatment trials will await their completion.

Depressive Symptomatology

Many women experienced high levels of depressive symptoms even though they did not meet the Research Diagnostic Criteria for major or minor depression. These were women who reported feeling sad, discouraged about the future, guilty, self-critical, irritable, tired; having problems sleeping and eating; and losing interest in other people. Although these women did not show the same degree of impairment as women who suffered from a major depression, and although these symptoms may not have been present on a daily basis, these symptoms can be very distressing and reduce a woman's ability to function effectively at home and on the job and can often impair a woman's relationships with her family and friends. This perspective is underscored by the very significant correlations between our measure of overall social adjustment (the SAS-SR) and the 2 depression measures (BDI, SCL-90-R depression subscale) at 3, 6, and 9 weeks postpartum. It is for these reasons that attention to changes in level of symptomatic depression is so important and why it is necessary to understand the correlates and predictors of elevated levels of symptomatic depression.

Demographic Variables

Surprisingly, none of the sociodemographic variables showed any associations with levels of symptomatic depression at 3, 6, or 9 weeks postpartum. Even among the nonchildbearing women, the only significant finding was that younger age was associated with higher levels of symptomatic depression at 3 weeks postpartum. These findings suggest that, at least among residents of a mixed urban, suburban, rural county in the Midwest, indices of relative social disadvantage are not particularly associated with higher levels of symptomatic depression. Although this sample was not as heterogeneous as some (e.g., O'Hara et al., 1982), it was composed of women who were recruited from private practices and a public clinic in equal proportions. Sociodemographic factors also were not associated with syndromal postpartum depression, a relatively consistent finding in the literature. Together, these findings suggest that relative social disadvantage is not a significant factor in explaining any element of a postpartum depressive experience.

Psychopathology Variables

Several indices of psychopathology were associated with higher levels of symptomatic depression at 3, 6, and 9 weeks postpartum. These indices included number of past episodes of depression, depressed first-degree relative, history of premenstrual major depression, and the postpartum blues. Needless to say, level of symptomatic depression during pregnancy was also associated with level of symptomatic depression after delivery. All of these findings point to the important role that past episodes of affective disorder and depression in the family play in driving future dysphoric mood.

Social and Cognitive Variables

Although social support was not associated with increased risk for syndromal depression after delivery, lower levels of social support were associated with higher levels of symptomatic depression 3, 6, and 9 weeks after delivery. In particular, women who reported less overall satisfaction with the support they were receiving during pregnancy and women who were less satisfied with the support provided by their partner after delivery had higher levels of symptomatic depression at each of the postpartum assessments. These findings also correspond to the findings of lower levels of marital satisfaction and adjustment among women with higher levels of symptomatic depression at 6 and 9 weeks postpartum. Overall, these results once again point to the importance of the marital relationship and the behavior of the spouse in the woman's affective state. Women who are happy in the marriage and feel supported by the spouse are much less likely to be experiencing high levels of symptomatic depression.

Our single measure of cognitive vulnerability, the Self-Control Questionnaire (Rehm et al., 1981), was not associated with syndromal depression; however, higher levels of dysfunctional self-control beliefs measured during pregnancy were associated with higher levels of symptomatic depression 6 and 9 weeks after delivery. Moreover, in the hierarchical multiple regression predicting level of symptomatic depression at 9 weeks postpartum, the conjunction of high levels of dysfunctional self-control beliefs and high levels of negative life events was a significant predictor over and above the main effects of the 2 variables. Lewinsohn et al. (1988) had argued that cognitive vulnerability factors such as dysfunctional self-control beliefs were uniquely predictive of symptomatic depression level. That is, dysfunctional self-control beliefs increase the likelihood of the negative affect tapped by measures like the Beck Depression Inventory but do not directly increase the likelihood of syndromal depression. For example, within the self-control theory of depression, it is posited that depression-prone individuals attend to negative events and negative outcomes of their own behavior, set high standards for their own conduct, unnecessarily blame themselves for failure, and provide little self-reward and excessive self-punishment. This dysfunctional self-regulatory process is hypothesized to increase an individual's risk for both depression symptoms and syndromal depression (Rehm, 1977). Our findings from this and an earlier study (O'Hara et al., 1984) suggest that dysfunctional self-control beliefs do increase risk for high levels of symptomatic depression but not for syndromal depression.

Stressors

Number of negative life events in the third trimester of pregnancy and number of childcare-related stressors early in the puerperium were both consistently associated with level of symptomatic depression at 3, 6, and 9 weeks postpartum. In addition to an interaction with self-control beliefs (described above), there were 2 other significant interactions that involved negative events. Both number of childcare-related stressors by prepartum syndromal depression and number of negative life events by prepartum syndromal depression were significant in predicting level of symptomatic depression at 9 weeks postpartum. These findings suggest that both the main effects of stress variables and their interaction with vulnerability factors are important in understanding risk for high levels of postpartum symptomatic depression.

In summary, poor postpartum adjustment as reflected by the Beck Depression Inventory and the SCL-90-R depression subscale was largely the continuation of poor adjustment during pregnancy or before. Factors that may improve or diminish a woman's social adjustment after childbirth include the occurrence of stressful life events and the social support provided to her during pregnancy and after delivery by her spouse, parents, and confidants. In a practical sense, it is important to recognize that a woman's functioning during pregnancy will be a good predictor of her functioning after delivery; and that changes in her social environment, some of which may be controllable (e.g., help from spouse or others) and some of which may be uncontrollable (e.g., occurrence of negative life event) may change the trajectory of a woman's social adjustment after delivery, for better or worse.

Postpartum Blues

The postpartum blues is a real phenomenon. We found, as have many other investigators, clear evidence of a peaking of dysphoric mood after delivery between days 4 and 8 (Iles et al., 1989; Kendell et al., 1984; Levy, 1987; O'Hara et al., 1990). There is no evidence that nonchildbearing women show any such pattern associated with a friend's delivery (O'Hara et al., 1990) or that women undergoing a nonobstetrical surgical procedure show this pattern (Kendell et al., 1984; Levy, 1987). In this section we will comment on issues of measurement, the comparability of our findings to other studies regarding prevalence of the blues, and issues relevant to causal factors.

Measurement and Prevalence

The postpartum blues has generally been defined as an affective disturbance of mild severity that occurs sometime during the first week or so postpartum (Kennerley & Gath, 1989a; O'Hara, Schlechte, Lewis, & Wright, 1991; Stein, 1982; Yalom et al., 1968). However, there has been little agreement on how the blues should be measured. In fact, we defined and measured the blues in *three* different ways in the current study. The Pitt (1973) criteria of the presence of both significant tearfulness and low mood is one definition of the blues that puts primary emphasis on crying or tearfulness (Yalom et al., 1968). The Pitt criteria were assessed in the context of the 9-week postpartum interview and yielded the highest estimate of prevalence, 42%. This estimate was similar to or somewhat below other studies that used identical or similar criteria. For example, 40% of women met criteria in Condon and Watson (1987), 50% of women met criteria in Pitt (1973), and 67% of women met similar criteria in Yalom et al. (1968). The Handley criteria (Handley et al., 1980), which were also assessed in the context of the 9-week postpartum interview, were more stringent than the Pitt criteria and demanded the presence of at least 4 of 7 symptoms to at least a mild degree. Again, similar to the case for the Pitt criteria, our rates of the blues were comparable to rates that had been reported in earlier studies. Our rate for the Handley criteria of 26% was comparable to an Icelandic study (Halldorsdottir, 1989) that used the Stein Blues Questionnaire (Stein, 1980) and obtained a prevalence rate of 28%; and to a German study (Lanczik et al., 1992) that obtained a prevalence rate of 28%, based on patient subjective report. Finally, we defined the blues on the basis of Visual Analogue Scales (Kendell et al., 1981; Kendell et al., 1984). Subjects whose scores were among the highest 26% (the percentage of childbearing subjects meeting Handley criteria) on days 4, 6, and 8 postpartum met the VAS criteria for the blues. This approach, of course, determined the percentage of women meeting VAS Blues criteria. However, the strength of the VAS assessment was that it occurred in the first week postpartum. The Pitt and the Handley criteria were assessed retrospectively. Unfortunately, there was little in our findings to recommend one of our blues measures over the others. Finally, it should be noted that the best validated blues measure yielded a blues prevalence of between 42% and 60% (Kennerley & Gath, 1989a). Unfortunately, that measure was unavailable when the current study was undertaken. In sum, our findings and those of earlier studies suggest that, depending upon how the blues is defined, the prevalence rate may range from about 25% to about 75%.

Causal Factors

The blues has often been regarded as a hormonally driven consequence of childbearing and a great deal of research has been undertaken to test various hormonal hypotheses (Kennerley & Gath, 1986; O'Hara, 1987). Two major reasons for this perspective are that the blues is quite common, and that the first week postpartum is a time of dramatic and rapid changes in levels of steroid hormones such as the estrogens, progesterone, and cortisol, and peptide hormones such as prolactin (George & Sandler, 1988). The blues is so common that it may simply be a normal response to a very positive but physically demanding event (i.e., childbirth) (Kennerley & Gath, 1986; Yalom et al., 1968). That is, the blues may simply reflect the "letdown" that some women feel after a long and sometimes difficult pregnancy, which culminates in the excitement and satisfaction of childbirth. This process of reestablishing normal function and daily routines requires physical, psychological, and social adjustments, part of which may be reflected in brief periods in which emotional equilibrium is shaken. A second perspective is that the blues is within the spectrum of affective disorders and represents a minor and short-lasting negative affective response to childbirth in women who show typical vulnerabilities for affective disorder (Kennerley & Gath, 1986; O'Hara, Schlechte, Lewis, & Wright, 1991).

The prepartum and postpartum factors that were predictive of or associated with our various indices of the blues would suggest that the blues falls within the realm of affective disorders. For example, women who experienced the blues had higher levels of depressive symptomatology during pregnancy, had more past depressions, and were more likely to have had a diagnosis of cyclothymia and premenstrual major depression than women who did not experience the blues. These findings were in contrast to the findings of the best previous prospective study of the blues (Kennerley & Gath, 1989b), which found no evidence that past history of affective disorder was associated with the blues; however, consistent with our results, Kennerley and Gath did find that depressive symptomatology measured during pregnancy was associated with the blues. One major difference between Kennerley and Gath and the current study was that they used "treatment" as the criterion for a previous depression, whereas we used the Research Diagnostic Criteria to determine the presence of previous episodes of depression. It is likely that many of their subjects who had not received treatment for depression in the past had experienced an untreated depressive episode. No other study of the blues to date has included such a formal assessment of past personal and family history of depression; however, other studies using less rigorous assessments of past depression have obtained findings consistent with our own (Stein, 1980; Yalom et al., 1968). In sum, emotional adjustment during pregnancy and previous history of depression show a clear relation to the blues and support the possible link between affective disorder and the postpartum blues (Kennerley & Gath, 1986).

The major social stressors associated with the blues were negative life events occurring in the second trimester of pregnancy (but not the third trimester) and childcare-related stressors. Why negative events in the second trimester would be associated with the blues is unclear, particularly in the absence of any association between third-trimester negative events and the blues. It was speculated in chapter 7 that two possibilities were that there was a delayed effect of the negative events or that it was a chance finding. This last interpretation is supported by Kennerley and Gath's (1989b) findings of no significant associations between negative life events (assessed in a similar manner) in the second or third trimesters and the presence of the blues.

Childcare-related stressors tend to be smaller events that may occur frequently or over an extended period and are similar to the "unpleasant events" described by Lewinsohn et al. (1979). In earlier work we had found that smaller unpleasant events tended to be associated with daily mood (O'Hara & Rehm, 1979). The childcare-related stressors probably tap important current concerns of recently delivered women and have a significant impact on mood. The other major negative events that occurred within a few days of the occurrence of the blues for some women were obstetric stressors. Interestingly, neither obstetric stressors, in general, nor the occurrence of a cesarean section, in particular, were associated with the blues. The lack of findings for obstetrical variables was in accord with Kennerley and Gath (1989b). However, the earlier literature has been quite mixed with respect to the role of obstetrical factors in the blues (Ballinger, Buckley, Naylor, & Stansfield, 1979; Davidson, 1972; Pitt, 1973; Yalom et al., 1968). It may be that it is the women's appraisal of the significance of the obstetric stressors more than the actual events that determines the impact on mood in the early puerperium.

There was some indication (though not strong) that the experience of social support during pregnancy and women's expectations of support after delivery were associated with the occurrence of the blues. We did not specifically assess social support perceived by women during the first week after delivery. However, 2 items from the Childcare Stress Inventory targeted lack of attention and help from the husband, experiences reported by between 29% and 36% of women. These experiences were rated as relatively distressing, and the "attention from husband" variable was associated with the blues defined by Handley and Pitt criteria. However, neither variable was significantly associated with the blues based on the VAS criteria. Future studies will need to incorporate measures of social support, particularly from the spouse, into the early postpartum assessments in order more adequately to assess the association between lack of social support and the blues.

There was very little support in our study for any of the hormonal hypotheses. However, levels of free and total estriol were more elevated during late pregnancy and the early puerperium in women who experienced the blues than in women who did not experience the blues. Also, women who experienced the blues evidenced a greater drop in free estriol from the end of pregnancy to day 1 postpartum than women who did not experience the blues. The estrogen hypothesis would predict that estrogen levels would be relatively low after delivery. Our findings of higher levels of estriol during late pregnancy and the greater drop in estriol levels after delivery were consistent with the estrogen hypothesis (Steiner, 1979). Nevertheless, we did not find that postpartum levels of any of the estrogens were lower in women who experienced the blues. Overall, our data do suggest the possibility that the relative levels of pre- and postpartum estrogen may be more important than the absolute levels of postpartum estrogen in putting women at risk for the blues. In the only two previous studies that have found significant effects for estrogens, one reported lower levels of prepartum estrogen and one reported higher levels of postpartum estrogen in women who experienced the blues (Feksi et al., 1984; Nott et al., 1976). The findings of neither of the earlier studies provide much support for the estrogen withdrawal hypothesis, and our study provides only modest support.

Pregnancy

When our group initially began work on the problem of postpartum depression in 1979, we were faced with the problem of when during pregnancy we should establish a baseline against which to judge changes in mood and social adjustment that occurred after delivery. The literature was not entirely clear, but it seemed that the second trimester might be desirable. During the first trimester, women frequently experience morning sickness and fatigue; and during the third trimester, the fullness of pregnancy (i.e., nearly full size of fetus and its effects of sleep, bladder control, energy, etc.) might have effects on mood that would be relatively negative. What we found, of course, was that with respect to indices of depressive mood and social adjustment, both the second and third trimesters are associated with significantly poorer adjustment than practically any time after delivery. These findings have been replicated again and again, particularly in North American studies that have tracked symptomatic depression and social adjustment over pregnancy and the puerperium (Elliott et al., 1983; Gotlib et al., 1989; O'Hara et al., 1982; O'Hara et al., 1984; O'Hara et al., 1990; Troutman & Cutrona, 1990). It is clear that at least part of the higher levels of symptomatic depression and lower levels of social adjustment is due to somatic discomfort, which is common during pregnancy. The somatic discomfort scale of the BDI reaches very high levels late in pregnancy and slowly normalizes after delivery, reaching normal levels by nine weeks postpartum. However, somatic discomfort does not necessarily explain why some women suffer more than others and why some women experience syndromal depression during pregnancy, a time during which the onset of serious psychopathology is relatively uncommon (Kendell et al., 1987).

In contrast to the case for postpartum syndromal and symptomatic depression, social disadvantage was associated with both syndromal and symptomatic depression in pregnant women. Indices such as lower educational attainment by the spouse, not working during pregnancy, and lower socioeconomic status were associated with increased risk for syndromal depression during pregnancy and, for several of these variables, with increased risk of high levels of depressive symptomatology. Similar findings of an association between social disadvantage and depression during pregnancy but not after delivery have been obtained in earlier studies (Cox et al., 1982; Gotlib et al., 1991). Why these indices of social disadvantage would be associated with depression during pregnancy but not with depression after delivery is not clear. Perhaps being relatively social disadvantaged during pregnancy led to more negative expectations regarding the family's ability to cope financially with a new baby. These negative expectations/worries might have reoriented a woman's attention during pregnancy away from the positive aspects of motherhood and toward the problems and difficulties that would be occasioned by the birth of the baby. This negative cognitive set may have been, in part, responsible for some of the depressive symptoms experienced by these pregnant women.

Several psychopathology risk factors were related to syndromal and symptomatic depression during pregnancy. Past histories of depression and alcoholism were both associated with syndromal and symptomatic depression, and history of alcoholism in the partner was associated with higher levels of symptomatic depression during the second and third trimesters. The findings regarding the women's psychiatric history are similar to those obtained in two studies conducted in London (Kumar & Robson, 1984; Zajicek, 1981) and mirror what has been observed about the role of past psychopathology in predicting depression after delivery. However, the findings regarding the association between partners' alcoholism and symptomatic depression during pregnancy were the only ones to implicate partner psychopathology as being a potential factor in syndromal or symptomatic depression or the blues among the childbearing women. Although it would seem sensible that having a partner who had a history of abusing alcohol would lead to higher levels of symptomatic depression, it is not clear why this should be observed for women during pregnancy but not after delivery. One possibility, of course, is that the alcohol-abusing spouse may decrease abusive drinking behavior for a period of time after the baby is born. Unfortunately, we did not collect data of that sort. Spouse psychiatric history was investigated in one other study, and it was found to be associated with postpartum rather than pregnancy depression and anxiety (Kumar & Robson, 1984).

There was a consistent theme for the childbearing women that social support from the partner was not adequate. This finding held for both syndromal and symptomatic depression. Also, relative lack of parental support was associated with higher levels of symptomatic depression during pregnancy. Finally, overall dissatisfaction with support during pregnancy was associated with both syndromal and symptomatic depression. These findings were in contrast to the findings for the role of social support, particularly from the spouse, in postpartum syndromal depression.

With respect to cognitive constructs, dysfunctional self-control beliefs were associated with both syndromal and symptomatic depression. Higher levels of negative life events were also associated with both syndromal and symptomatic depression.

Future Directions

This volume has been primarily concerned with the causes of postpartum depression and secondarily concerned with its consequences. In chapter 1 it was briefly noted that there is a literature that suggests that women who experience postpartum depression are likely to be at continuing risk for future depressions and that their children may suffer as well. These findings have been echoed in our own work (see Chapter 2; Philipps & O'Hara, 1991). Despite the important consequences of postpartum depression, relatively little work has been done to systematically identify and intervene with women at risk (see Chapter 1). Barriers to work in this area include the difficulty of determining reasonably sensitive, specific, and objective risk factors for postpartum depression and the general lack of recognition in obstetrical settings of the importance of identifying women at risk for poor psychological adjustment after delivery. All of these considerations lead to suggestions for future research, including (1) long-term follow-up of postpartum depressed mothers and their family; (2) prevention and treatment research; and (3) the development of protocols for identifying and monitoring women at risk and for treating women who become depressed.

Long-Term Consequences of Postpartum Depression

As noted in chapter 1, several studies have followed community samples of childbearing women and their children over several years. In general, these studies found that postpartum-depressed women and their children were at risk for future depressions in the case of the mothers and behavioral and/or cognitive problems in the case of the children (e.g., Kumar & Robson, 1984; Ghodsian et al., 1984; Philipps & O'Hara, 1991). However, the absolute number of postpartum-depressed women included in these samples has been relatively small because the depressed women make up only 10% to 15% of the childbearing sample followed over time. It is important to identify a large sample of postpartum-depressed women after delivery and follow them and their children prospectively to determine long-term consequences for maternal functioning, family life, and the adjustment of the child (Campbell et al., 1992). Although the postpartum depressions may remit within a few months, residual deficits may continue and subsequent depressions may develop, as previous studies have suggested (see Chapter 1; Philipps & O'Hara, 1991).

Prevention and Treatment

The few studies that evaluated preventive and treatment interventions have demonstrated positive effects for childbearing women (Elliott et al., 1988; Holden et al., 1989). For example, relatively brief interventions during pregnancy with low- and high-risk women result in relatively lower levels of depressive symptomatology after delivery (Elliott et al., 1988; Gordon & Gordon, 1960). Brief client-centered counseling has also demonstrated effectiveness for postpartum depressed patients (Holden et al., 1989). Although the results of this work are promising, new studies should be undertaken using American samples and evaluating interventions that have demonstrated efficacy with nonpostpartum depression such as interpersonal psychotherapy and cognitive therapy (Beck et al., 1979; Elkin et al., 1989; Klerman, Weissman, Rounsaville, & Chevron, 1984). In addition, preventive interventions involving brief versions of interpersonal psychotherapy or cognitive therapy might be used with women at high risk for a postpartum depression as evidenced by past history of recurrent depression.

Identifying and Monitoring High-Risk Women

Routine obstetrical care does not usually include identifying women who may be at risk for postpartum depression or psychosis. Fortunately, the vast majority of women experience no significant depression after delivery; however, up to 10% of women experience a nonpsychotic depression; and about 1 in 1,000 women experience psychosis, often in the context of a manic or depressive episode. Many of these women have characteristics that can be identified during pregnancy and set the stage for more or less intensive monitoring for the first signs of a developing depression. During pregnancy women might be classified into 1 of 3 risks for depression categories: very high risk, high risk, and low risk.

The very-high-risk group includes women who are mentally ill at the time they become pregnant. Many of these women will already be in treatment, often under the care of a psychiatrist (Cohen, Heller, & Rosenbaum, 1989). Also included are women who have experienced a previous psychotic episode, which may or may not have been associated with childbirth, and women who have a history of bipolar depression. Some of these women will also be under the care of a mental health professional, but certainly not all of them. These women will come to the attention of the obstetrics staff through self-identification, communication from the treating mental health professional, or through screening done during a prenatal visit. Very-high-risk women may be monitored during pregnancy and puerperium by their mental health care providers. For women not in treatment, it may be necessary to use a screening measure, such as the Edinburgh Postnatal Depression Scale (Cox et al., 1987), that can be completed on a periodic basis during pregnancy and after delivery. Alternatively, obstetrics staff could assess symptoms of depression at the time of prenatal visits. The key element for these very-high-risk women would be to institute prophylactic treatment immediately after delivery (Robinson, Stewart, & Flak, 1986) or to begin treatment at the first sign of a developing depression. These treatments might involve a wide range of psychopharmacological and psychotherapeutic interventions (see Chapter 1; Robinson et al., 1986). Research on the effectiveness of prophylaxis and early intervention with very-high-risk women is only now beginning (Kumar, 1991).

The high-risk group includes women with a history of recurrent depressions, a history of anxiety disorder (e.g., panic, obsessive-compulsive disorder), and women with a strong family history of depression (O'Hara et al., 1984; O'Hara, Schlechte, Lewis, & Varner, 1991; Sichel, Cohen, Dimmock, & Rosenbaum, 1993). For these women postpartum depression is not an invariable consequence of delivery, but risk is greatly increased relative to women who do not have these characteristics. These women can be identified during pregnancy in very much the same way as women in the very-high-risk group; however, they are much less likely to be in treatment already. Moreover, if they have not ever been treated for their depressive or anxiety disorder, some more assessment, such as a brief, semistructured interview, may be required to identify these women (O'Hara et al., 1990; O'Hara, Schlechte, Lewis, & Varner, 1991).

The purpose of monitoring high-risk women is to identify and intervene early in a developing depression. Monitoring high-risk women would be similar to monitoring very-high-risk women. Periodic completion of the Edinburgh Postnatal Depression Scale or brief assessments conducted by obstetrics staff may be sufficient to detect the early stages of a postpartum depression. Interventions may include antidepressant medication and psychotherapeutic interventions. Some women, particularly if they have never been in treatment, may prefer a referral to a postpartum support group (see *PSI News*). Once again, very little work has been done to evaluate the effectiveness and efficiency of identifying, monitoring, and treating high-risk women. Work in this area should benefit the health and welfare of childbearing women and their families.

Summary

Since the time that the project reported in this volume began, there has been an explosion in research on postpartum depression, particularly in the areas of causes and consequences. Much has been learned about the relative prevalence of postpartum depression, its etiology, and the effects that it has on the functioning and welfare of women and children. The major tasks for the future are to prevent these depressive episodes when possible and, if necessary, to intervene early in the process. In order to accomplish these tasks, it will be necessary to develop sensitive and specific screening measures, educate obstetricians and nurses about postpartum depression, validate specific treatments for postpartum depression, and develop ways to reduce the negative effects of maternal depression on newborns and older children. It is to be hoped that these tasks will be accomplished in the next decade.

Appendix A
Childcare Stress Inventory*

Part I:

Below is a list of experiences you may have had since entering the hospital to deliver your baby. *Please indicate which of these events you experienced by circling the number of the event.* If you didn't experience the event, do not circle its number.

______ 1. Labor and/or delivery did not go the way you had hoped.
______ 2. Negative experience with hospital staff or hospital procedures.
______ 3. Conflict over childcare with family or friends.
______ 4. Strain in relationship with husband.
______ 5. Can't give enough time to husband.
______ 6. Not receiving enough support or attention from husband.
______ 7. Husband doesn't help with work as much as you would like.
______ 8. Overwhelmed by demands of infant care.
______ 9. House is more disorganized than usual.
______ 10. Problems feeding baby.
______ 11. Can't quiet baby's cries.
______ 12. Can't relax with baby.
______ 13. Baby has health problems.
______ 14. Concern that it is taking longer than you expected to learn to love the baby.
______ 15. Having trouble establishing regular feeding times.
______ 16. Having trouble establishing regular nap times and bed time for baby.
______ 17. Don't know what baby needs when he or she cries.
______ 18. Baby rarely or never seems content.
______ 19. Feel trapped or confined.
______ 20. Miss previous activities or work.

---

*Adapted with the permission of the developer, Carolyn E. Cutrona, 1994.

Part II:

Going back to the list of events in Part I, please use the lines in front of your circled numbers to rate how upsetting each event was for you. On a scale from 0 to 100, put a number that best reflects your distress. 0 will correspond with *not upsetting* and 100 would be *extremely upsetting*. If you didn't circle the number, do not rate it.

Part III:

Please list any other upsetting events you experienced that were related to having a new baby.

______ 21. ____.
______ 22. ____.
______ 23. ____.
______ 24. ____.

Please rate these events (if any) as in Part II.

Appendix B
Peripartum Events Scale*

Patient name ____

(___ ___ - ___ ___ ___ ___ ___)
Patient hospital number

(___ ___ - ___ ___ - ___ ___)
Date of delivery by month, date, year

(___ ___ - ___ ___ ___ ___ ___)
Infant hospital number

1. Demographic—2 is maximum — (11)
   a. Age <18 or >35
   b. Unmarried
   c. Less than HS education

2. Past obstetric history—all count equally — (12)
   a. Previous cesarean section, other uterine or cervical surgery, or uterine anomalies
   b. Previous perinatal death or SIDS
   c. Previous baby with congenital anomaly, mental retardation, or seizures
   d. Previous malpresentation, obstetric hemorrhage, positive Coombs test, or toxemia
   e. Three or more abortions
   f. Previous abnormally sized infants (LGA or SGA)
   g. Previous preterm (<37 weeks) or postterm (>41 weeks) delivery
   h. Less than 1 year since previous delivery

---

*This material first appeared in the Journal of Reproductive and Infant Psychology (1986) 4:95–97.

3. Medical risk factors—all count equally — (13)
   a. Hypertension
   b. Heart disease
   c. Endocrine disease, incl. diabetes
   d. Kidney disease
   e. Pulmonary disease
   f. Gastrointestinal disease
   g. Seizure disorder
   h. Anemia (Hgb <9.0)
   i. Extremes of pre-pregnant weight (<45 or >90 kg)
   j. Chemical abuse
   k. Other medical problems (0–1–2)

4. Obstetric risk factors—all count equally — (14)
   a. Abnormal weight gain (<4 kg or >18 kg)
   b. Abnormal uterine size, incl. multiple pregnancy
   c. Pre-eclampsia
   d. Significant bleeding
   e. Abnormal presentation
   f. Fever in labor
   g. Meconium-stained amniotic fluid

5. Indication for admission to labor and delivery — (15)
   a. Ruptured membranes >12 hours without labor
   b. Vaginal bleeding
   c. Decreased fetal movement
   d. Pain other than labor
   e. Premature labor (<37 weeks) or postdates labor (>41 weeks)
   f. Infection
   g. Indicated induction of labor (ex. postdates)
   h. Previous cesarean section, in labor
   i. Other (0–1–2)

6. Progress in labor — (16)
   a. Precipitous (<3 hours)
   b. Secondary arrest of labor requiring oxytocin
   c. Secondary arrest of labor requiring pelvimetry
   d. Requiring more than 3 analgesics during labor
   e. Other (0–1–2)

7. Method of delivery — (17)
   a. Midforceps
   b. Vaginal breech
   c. Cesarean section—primary cesarean section (2 points)
   d. Repeat cesarean section (1 point)

   e. Vaginal multiple gestation
   f. Other (0–1–2)

8. Duration of labor — (18)
   a. First stage
      1. Primigravidas (>20 hours)
      2. Multigravidas (>14 hours)
   b. Second stage
      1. Primigravidas (>2 hours)
      2. Multigravidas (>1 ½ hours)
   c. Third stage >30 minutes

9. Fetal monitoring — (19)
   a. Electronic fetal heart rate monitoring (internal or external)*
   b. Abnormal fetal heart rate monitoring
   c. Electronic contraction monitoring (internal or external)*
   d. Abnormal contraction monitoring
   e. Fetal blood sampling performed
   f. Abnormal fetal blood sampling (2 points)

10. Delivery complications — (20)
    a. Blood loss >600 cc
    b. Significant lacerations
    c. Puerperal infection
    d. Anesthetic complications
    e. Manual removal of placenta
    f. Other (0–1)

11. Infant outcome — (21)
    a. <37 weeks or >41 weeks
    b. SGA or LGA
    c. One-minute Apgar <6
    d. Five-minute Apgar <8
    e. Neonatal complications
       1. Need for pH correction
       2. Need for volume expansion
       3. Need for transfusion or exchange transfusion
       4. Hypoglycemia
       5. Hyperbilirubinemia
       6. Hypocalcemia
       7. Treatment for sepsis
       8. Meconium aspiration pneumonitis
       9. Other (0–1–2)

---

*If both FHR and contractions are monitored, *both* should be noted.

Comments: ____

Appendix C
Social Support Interview*

A. Support available from confidant, parent, and spouse

1. Is there anyone in particular you confide in or talk to about yourself or your problems? (Ask for first name of person.) Yes—1; No—2
   Name: ____________ —
2. Which of your parents are you most able to confide in and talk to about yourself and your problems? Mother—1; Father—2 —

I would like to ask you some questions about your relationship with confidant (name), parent (mother or father), and husband (partner).

Questions 3–12, Confidant, parent and spouse

3. Can you rely on this person for help in *doing things* when you may need it, such as assisting on the job, helping with household tasks, providing personal or family care (e.g., babysitting), or even lending money?
   1—No
   2—Rarely
   3—Sometimes
   4—Usually
   5—Always
   8—Don't know
   9—No person

   a. Confidant —
   b. Parent —
   c. Spouse —

*Adapted with permission of the developer, Daniel P. Mueller, 1994.

4. Can you turn to this person for emotional support when you need it?
   1—No
   2—Rarely
   3—Sometimes
   4—Usually
   5—Always
   8—Don't know
   9—No person

   a. Confidant —
   b. Parent —
   c. Spouse —

5. Can this person rely on you for help in *doing things* when he/she may need it, such as assisting on the job, helping with household tasks, providing personal or family care (e.g., babysitting) or even lending money?
   1—No
   2—Rarely
   3—Sometimes
   4—Usually
   5—Always
   9—No person

   a. Confidant —
   b. Parent —
   c. Spouse —

6. Can this person turn to you for *emotional support* when he/she may need it?
   1—No
   2—Rarely
   3—Sometimes
   4—Usually
   5—Always
   9—No person

   a. Confidant —
   b. Parent —
   c. Spouse —

7. In general, over the past year, has your association with this person made your life easier (or more enjoyable) or more difficult (or more burdensome)?
   1—Much easier/enjoyable
   2—Slightly easier/enjoyable
   3—Neither easier nor more difficult
   4—Slightly more difficult/burdensome
   5—Much more difficult/burdensome
   9—No person

   a. Confidant —
   b. Parent —
   c. Spouse —

8. When you have problems or troubles, do you talk them over with this person?
   1—Always
   2—Usually

   a. Confidant —
   b. Parent —

3—Sometimes c. Spouse —
4—Rarely
5—Never
9—No person

9. Do you feel free to talk about anything you wish with this person?
1—Very free a. Confidant —
2—Somewhat free b. Parent —
3—Moderately free c. Spouse —
4—Not very free
5—Not at all free
9—No person

10. Does this person tell you about his/her problems?
1—Always a. Confidant —
2—Usually b. Parent —
3—Sometimes c. Spouse —
4—Rarely
5—Never
9—No person

11. Is this person there when you need him/her?
1—Always a. Confidant —
2—Usually b. Parent —
3—Sometimes c. Spouse —
4—Rarely
5—Never
9—No person

12. Do you anticipate being able to rely on this person for help with childcare after your baby is born?
1—All of the time a. Confidant —
2—Frequently b. Parent —
3—About half the time c. Spouse —
4—Occasionally
5—Never
9—No person

B. General availability and use of support

1. In general, do you feel there is someone you can turn to in times of need? —
1—Always

2—Usually
3—Sometimes
4—Rarely
5—Never

2. Are you ever hesitant (or reluctant) to ask for help from family and/or friends when you may need it? —
1—Always
2—Usually
3—Sometimes
4—Rarely
5—Never

3. Generally speaking, when you may need help in doing something, or advice, information, support, etc., do you turn to the people available to you? —
1—Always
2—Usually
3—Sometimes
4—Rarely
5—Never
8—Not applicable, no one available

4. In general, how satisfied are you with the help/support provided by the people available to you? —
1—Very satisfied
2—Somewhat satisfied
3—Neither satisfied or dissatisfied
4—Somewhat dissatisfied
5—Very dissatisfied
8—Not applicable, has no one available or does not use them

References

Abramson, L.Y., Seligman, M.E.P., & Teasdale, J.D. (1978). Learned helplessness in humans: Critique and reformulation. *Journal of Abnormal Psychology, 87,* 49–74.

Achenbach, T.M. (1978). The child behavior profile: I. Boys aged 6–11. *Journal of Consulting and Clinical Psychology, 46,* 478–488.

Achenbach, T.M., & Edelbrock, C.S. (1979). The child behavior profile: II. Boys aged 12–16 and girls aged 6–11 and 12–16. *Journal of Consulting and Clinical Psychology, 47,* 223–233.

Achenbach, T.M., & Edelbrock, C.S. (1983). *Manual for the child behavior checklist and revised child behavior profile.* Burlington, VT: Department of Psychiatry, University of Vermont.

American Psychiatric Association (1968). *Diagnostic and statistical manual of mental disorders* (2nd ed.). Washington, DC: American Psychiatric Association.

American Psychiatric Association (1980). *Diagnostic and statistical manual of mental disorders* (3rd ed.). Washington, DC: American Psychiatric Association.

American Psychiatric Association (1987). *Diagnostic and statistical manual of mental disorders* (3rd ed., rev.). Washington, DC: American Psychiatric Association.

Andreasen, N.C., Endicott, J., Spitzer, R.L., & Winokur, G. (1977). The family history methods using diagnostic criteria. *Archives of General Psychiatry, 34,* 1229–1235.

Atkinson, A.K., & Rickel, A.U. (1984). Postpartum depression in primiparous parents. *Journal of Abnormal Psychology, 93,* 115–119.

Ballinger, C.B., Kay, D.S.G., Naylor, G.J., & Smith, A.H.W. (1982). Some biochemical findings during pregnancy and after delivery in relation to mood change. *Psychological Medicine, 12,* 549–556.

Ballinger, C.B., Buckley, D.E., Naylor, G.J., & Stansfield, D.A. (1979). Emotional disturbance following childbirth: Clinical findings and urinary excretion of cyclic AMP (adenosine 3′5′ cyclic monophosphate). *Psychological Medicine, 9,* 293–300.

Bebbington, P., Hurry, J., Tennant, C., Sturt, E., & Wing, J.K. (1981). Epidemiology of mental disorders in Camberwell. *Psychological Medicine, 11,* 561–597.

Beck, A.T. (1970). *Depression: Causes and treatment.* Philadelphia: University of Pennsylvania Press.

Beck, A.T., Rush, A.J., Shaw, B.F., & Emery, G. (1979). *Cognitive therapy of depression.* New York: Guilford.

Beck, A.T., Ward, C.H., Mendelson, M., Mock, J., & Erbaugh, J. (1961). An inventory for measuring depression. *Archives of General Psychiatry, 4,* 561–569.

Belsher, G., & Costello, C.G. (1988). Relapse after recovery from unipolar depression: A critical review. *Psychological Bulletin, 104,* 84–96.

Belsky, J., Lang, M., & Rovine, M. (1985). Stability and change in marriage: A second study. *Journal of Marriage and the Family, 47,* 855–866.

Blair, R.A., Gilmore, J.S., Playfair, H.R., Tisdall, M.W., & O'Shea, M.W. (1970). Puerperal depression: A study of predictive factors. *Journal of the Royal College of General Practitioners, 19,* 22–25.

Blumberg, N.J. (1980). Effects of neonatal risk, maternal attitude, and cognitive style on early postpartum adjustment. *Journal of Abnormal Psychology, 89,* 139–150.

Bower, W.H., & Altschule, M.D. (1956). Use of progesterone in the treatment of postpartum psychosis. *New England Journal of Medicine, 254,* 157–162.

Braverman, J., & Roux, J.F. (1978). Screening for the patient at risk for postpartum depression. *Obstetrics and Gynecology, 52,* 731–736.

Breslau, N. (1985). Depressive symptoms, major depression, and genrealized anxiety: A comparison of self-reports on CES-D and results from diagnosis with interviews. *Psychiatry Research, 15,* 219–229.

Breslau, N., & Davis, G.C. (1986). Chronic stress and major depression. *Archives of General Psychiatry, 43,* 309–314.

Brinsmead, M., Smith, R., Singh, B., Lewin, T., & Owens, P. (1985). Peripartum concentrations of beta endorphin and cortisol and maternal mood states. *Australian and New Zealand Journal of Obstetrics and Gynecology, 25,* 194–197.

Brockington, I.F., Cernik, K.F., Schofield, E.M., Downing, A.R., Francis, A.F., & Keelan, C. (1981). Puerperal psychosis: Phenomena and diagnosis. *Archives of General Psychiatry, 38,* 829–833.

Brown, G.W., & Harris, T. (1978). *Social origins of depression: A study of psychiatric disorder in women.* New York: The Free Press.

Brown, G.W., & Harris, T. (1989). *Depression.* In G.W. Brown & T. Harris (Eds.), *Life events and illness* (pp. 49–93). New York: Guilford.

Cadoret, R.J., & Winokur, G. (1974). Depression in alcoholism. *Annals of the New York Academy of Sciences. 233,* 34–39.

Campbell, J.L., & Winokur, G. (1985). Post-partum affective disorders: Selected biological aspects. In D.G. Inwood (Ed.), *Recent advances in post-partum psychiatric disorders* (pp. 19–40). Washington, DC: American Psychiatric Press.

Campbell, S.B., & Cohn, J.F. (1991). Prevalence and correlates of postpartum depression in first-time mothers. *Journal of Abnormal Psychology, 100,* 594–599.

Campbell, S.B., Cohn, J.F., Flanagan, C., Popper, S., & Meyers, T. (1992). Course and correlates of postpartum depression during the transition to parenthood. *Development and Psychopathology, 4,* 29–47.

Carothers, A.D., & Murray, L. (1990). Estimating psychiatry morbidity by logistic regression: Application to post-natal depression in a community sample. *Psychological Medicine, 20,* 695–702.

Caplan, H.L., Cogill, S.R., Alexandra, H., Robson, K.M., Katz, R., & Kumar, R. (1989). Maternal depression and the emotional development of the child. *British Journal of Psychiatry, 154,* 818–822.

Carroll, B.J., & Steiner, M. (1978). The psychobiology of premenstrual dysphoria: The role of prolactin. *Psychoneuroendocrinology, 3,* 171–180.

Cogill, S.R., Caplan, H.L., Alexandra, H., Robson, K.M., & Kumar, R. (1986). Impact of maternal postnatal depression on cognitive development of young children. *British Medical Journal, 292,* 1165–1167.

Cohen, L.S., Heller, V.L., & Rosenbaum, J.F. (1989). Treatment guidelines for psychotropic drug use in pregnancy. *Psychosomatics, 30,* 25–33.

Cohen, N., Gotlieb, H., Kershner, J., & Wehrspann, W. (1985). Concurrent validity of internalizing and externalizing profile patterns of the Achenbach Child Behavior Checklist. *Journal of Consulting and Clinical Psychology, 53,* 724–728.

Cohn, J.F., Campbell, S.B., Matias, R., & Hopkins, J. (1990). Face-to-face interactions of postpartum depressed and nondepressed mother-infant pairs of 2 months. *Developmental Psychology, 26,* 15–23.

Condon, J.T., & Watson, T.L. (1987). The maternity blues: Exploration of a psychological hypothesis. *Acta Psychiatrica Scandinavica, 76,* 164–171.

Cooper, P.J., Campbell, E.A., Day, A., Kennerley, H., & Bond, A. (1988). Non-psychotic psychiatric disorder after childbirth: A prospective study of prevalence, incidence, course and nature. *British Journal of Psychiatry, 152,* 799–806.

Cox, J.L. (1983). Postnatal depression: A comparison of African and Scottish women. *Social Psychiatry, 18,* 25–28.

Cox, J.L., Connor, Y.M., Henderson, I., McGuire, R.J., & Kendell, R.E. (1983). Prospective study of the psychiatric disorders of childbirth by self-report questionnaire. *Journal of Affective Disorders, 5,* 1–7.

Cox, J.L., Connor, Y., & Kendell, R.E. (1982). Prospective study of the psychiatric disorders of childbirth. *British Journal of Psychiatry, 140,* 111–117.

Cox, J.L., Holden, J.M., & Sagovsky, R. (1987). Detection of postnatal depression: Development of the 10-item Edinburgh Postnatal Depression Scale. *British Journal of Psychiatry, 150,* 782–786.

Cox, J.L., Murray, D., & Chapman, G. (1993). A controlled study of the onset, duration and prevalence of postnatal depression. *British Journal of Psychiatry, 163,* 27–31.

Cox, J.L., Rooney, A., Thomas, P.F., & Wrate, R.W. (1984). How accurately do mothers recall postnatal depression? Further data from a 3 year follow-up study. *Journal of Psychosomatic Obstetrics and Gynaecology, 3,* 185–189.

Craighead, W.E., Hickey, K.S., & DeMonbreun, B.G. (1979). Distortion of perception of recall of neutral feedback in depression. *Cognitive Therapy and Research, 3,* 291–298.

Cutrona, C.E. (1983). Causal attributions and perinatal depression. *Journal of Abnormal Psychology, 92,* 161–172.

Cutrona, C.E. (1984). Social support and stress in the transition to parenthood. *Journal of Abnormal Psychology, 93,* 378–390.

Cytryn, L., McKnew, D.H., Zahn-Waxler, C., Radke-Yarrow, M., Gaensbauer, T.J., Harmon, R.J., & Lamour, M. (1984). A developmental view of affective disturbances in the children of affectively ill parents. *American Journal of Psychiatry, 141,* 219–222.

Dalton, K. (1971). Prospective study into puerperal depression. *British Journal of Psychiatry, 118,* 689–692.

Dalton, K. (1980). *Depression after childbirth.* Oxford: Oxford University Press.

Dalton, K. (1985). Progesterone prophylaxis used successfully in postnatal depression. *The Practitioner, 229,* 507–508.

Davidson, J.R.T. (1972). Post-partum mood changes in Jamaican women: A description and discussion of its significance. *British Journal of Psychiatry, 121,* 659–663.

Dean, C., & Kendell, R.E. (1981). The symptomatology of puerperal illnesses. *The British Journal of Psychiatry, 139,* 128–133.

DeLongis, A., Coyne, J.C., Dakof, G., Folkman, S., & Lazarus, R.S. (1982). Relationship of daily hassles, uplifts, and major life events to health status. *Health Psychology, 1,* 119–136.

Dennerstein, L., Morse, C.A., Varnavides, K. (1988). Premenstrual tension and depression—is there a relationship? *Journal of Psychosomatic Obstetrics and Gynaecology, 8,* 45–52.

Depue, R.A. (Ed.) (1979). *The psychobiology of the depressive disorders: Implications for the effects of stress.* New York: Academic Press.

Derogatis, L.R. (1983). *SCL-90-R: Administration, scoring, and procedures manual-II* (2nd ed.). Baltimore, MD: Clinical Psychometrics Research.

Dix, C. (1985). *The new mother syndrome: Coping with postpartum stress and depression.* Garden City, NY: Doubleday & Company.

Downey, G., & Coyne, J.C. (1990). Children of depressed parents: An integrative review. *Psychological Bulletin, 108,* 50–76.

Ehlert, U., Patalla, U., Kirschbaum, C., Piedmont, E., & Hellhammer, D.H. (1990). Postpartum blues: Salivary cortisol and psychological factors. *Journal of Psychosomatic Research, 34,* 319–325.

Elkin, I., Shea, M.T., Watkins, J.T., Imber, S.D., Sotsky, S.M., Collins, J.F., Glass, D.R., Pilkonis, P.A., Leber, W.R., Docherty, J.P., Fiester, S.J., & Parloff, M.B. (1989). National Institute of Mental Health Treatment of Depression Collaborative Research Program: General effectiveness of treatments. *Archives of General Psychiatry, 46,* 971–982.

Elliott, S.A., Rugg, A.J., Watson, J.P., & Brough, D.I. (1983). Mood changes during pregnancy and after the birth of a child. *British Journal of Clinical Psychology, 22,* 295–308.

Elliott, S.A., Sanjack, M., & Leverton, T.J. (1988). Parents groups in pregnancy: A preventive intervention for postnatal depression? In B.H. Gottlieb (Ed.), *Marshaling social support: Formats, processes, and effects* (pp. 87–110). Newbury Park, CA: Sage.

Endicott, J., Halbreich, U., Schacht, S., & Nee, J. (1981). Premenstrual changes and affective disorder. *Psychosomatic Medicine, 43,* 519–529.

Endicott, J., & Spitzer, R. (1978). A diagnostic interview: The Schedule for Affective Disorders and Schizophrenia. *Archives of General Psychiatry, 35,* 837–844.

Eysenck, H., & Eysenck, S.G.B. (1975). *Manual of the Eysenck Personality Questionnaire.* London: Hadder & Stoughton.

Feggetter, P., & Gath, D. (1981). Non-psychotic psychiatric disorders in women one year after childbirth. *Journal of Psychosomatic Research, 25,* 369–372.

Feksi, A., Harris, B., Walker, R.F., Riad-Fahmy, D., & Newcombe, R.G. (1984). "Maternity blues" and hormone levels in saliva. *Journal of Affective Disorders, 6,* 351–355.

Field, T., Healy, B., Goldstein, S., & Guthertz, M. (1990). Behavior-state matching and synchrony in mother-infant interactions of nondepressed versus depressed dyads. *Developmental Psychology, 26,* 7–14.

Field, T., Healy, B., Goldstein, S., Perry, S., Bendell, D., Schanberg, S., Zimmerman, E.A., & Kuhn, C. (1988). Infants of depressed mothers show "depressed" behavior even with nondepressed adults. *Child Development, 59,* 1569–1579.

Field, T., Sandberg, D., Garcia, R., Vega-Lahr, N., Goldstein, S., & Guy, L. (1985). Pregnancy problems, postpartum depression, and early mother-infant interactions. *Developmental Psychology, 21,* 1152–1156.

Fleming, A.S., Klein, E., & Corter, C. (1992). The effects of a social support group on depression, maternal attitudes and behavior in new mothers. *Journal of Child Psychology and Psychiatry, 33,* 685–698.

Gaensbauer, T.J., Harmon, R.J., Cytryn, L., & McKnew, D.H. (1984). Social and affective development in infants with a manic-depressive parent. *American Journal of Psychiatry, 141,* 223–229.

Gallagher, D., Thompson, L.W., & Levy, S.M. (1980). Clinical psychological assessment of older adults. In L.W. Poon (Ed.), *Aging in the 1980s* (pp. 19–40). Washington, DC: American Psychological Association.

Gard, P.R., Handley, S.L., Parsons, A.D., & Waldron, G. (1986). A multivariate investigation of postpartum mood disturbance. *British Journal of Psychiatry, 148,* 567–575.

Gelfand, D.M., & Teti, D.M. (1990). The effects of maternal depression on children. *Clinical Psychology Review, 10,* 329–353.

George, A.J., Copeland, J.R.M., & Wilson, K.C.M. (1980). Serum prolactin and the postpartum blues syndrome. *British Journal of Pharmacology, 70,* 102–103.

George, A., & Sandler, M. (1988). Endocrine and biochemical studies in puerperal mental disorders. In R. Kumar & I.F. Brockington (Eds.), *Motherhood and mental illness 2 Causes and consequences* (pp. 78–112). London: Wright.

George, A.J., & Wilson, K.C.M. (1983). Beta-endorphin and puerperal psychiatric symptoms. *British Journal of Pharmacology, 80,* 493P.

Ghodsian, M., Zajicek, E., & Wolkind, S. (1984). A longitudinal study of maternal depression and child behavior problems. *Journal of Child Psychology and Psychiatry and Allied Disciplines, 25,* 91–109.

Ghoneim, M.M., Hinrichs, J.V., O'Hara, M.W., Mehta, M.P., Pathak, D., Kumar, V., & Clark, C.R. (1988). Comparison of psychologic and cognitive functions after general or regional anesthesia. *Anesthesiology, 69,* 507–515.

Goldberg, D. (1972). *The detection of psychiatric illness by questionnaire.* London: Oxford University Press.

Gordon, R.E., & Gordon, K.K. (1960). Social factors in the prevention of postpartum emotional problems. *Obstetrics and Gynecology, 15,* 433–438.

Gotlib, I.H. (1984). Depression and general psychopathology in university students. *Journal of Abnormal Psychology, 93,* 19–30.

Gotlib, I.H., Whiffen, V.E., Mount, J.H., Milne, K., & Cordy, N.I. (1989). Prevalence rates and demographic characteristics associated with depression in pregnancy and the postpartum. *Journal of Consulting and Clinical Psychology, 57,* 269–274.

Gotlib, I.H., Whiffen, V.E., Wallace, P.M., & Mount, J.H. (1991). Prospective investigation of postpartum depression: Factors involved in onset and recovery. *Journal of Abnormal Psychology, 100,* 122–132.

Greenwood, J., & Parker, G. (1984). The dexamethasone suppression test in the puerperium. *Australian and New Zealand Journal of Psychiatry, 18,* 282–284.

Grimmell, K., & Larsen, V.L. (1965). Postpartum and depressive psychiatric symptoms and thyroid activity. *Journal of the American Medical Women's Association, 20,* 542–546.

Halbreich, U., Endicott, J., & Nee, J. (1982). The diversity of premenstrual changes as reflected in the Premenstrual Assessment Form. *Acta Psychiatric Scandinavica, 65,* 46–65.

Halldorsdottir, A. (1989). *Survey of post-partum blues in Iceland.* Unpublished manuscript. Icelandic School of Midwifery, Reykjavik.

Halonen, J.S., & Passman, R.H. (1985). Relaxation training and expectation in the treatment of postpartum distress. *Journal of Consulting and Clinical Psychology, 53,* 839–845.

Hamilton, J.A. (1962). *Postpartum psychiatric disorders.* St Louis, MO: The C.V. Mosby Co.

Hamilton, J.A., & Harberger, P.N. (Eds.) (1992). *Postpartum psychiatric illness: A picture puzzle.* Philadelphia, PA: University of Pennsylvania Press.

Hammen, C. (1991). *Depression runs in families: The social context of risk and resilience in children of depressed mothers.* New York: Springer-Verlag.

Handley, S.L., Dunn, T.L., Baker, J.M., Cockshott, C., & Gould, S. (1977). Mood changes in puerperium, and plasma tryptophan and cortisol concentrations. *British Medical Journal, 2,* 18–22.

Handley, S.L., Dunn, T.L., Waldron, G., & Baker, J.M. (1980). Tryptophan, cortisol and puerperal mood. *British Journal of Psychiatry, 136,* 498–508.

Hannah, P., Adams, D., Lee, A., Glover, V., & Sandler, M. (1992). Links between early post-partum mood and post-natal depression. *British Journal of Psychiatry, 160,* 777–780.

Harkness, S. (1987). The cultural mediation of postpartum depression. *Medical Anthropology Quarterly, 1,* 194–209.

Harris, B. (1980). Prospective trial of L-tryptophan in maternity blues. *British Journal of Psychiatry, 137,* 233–235.

Harris, B. (1981). "Maternity blues" in East African clinic attenders. *Archives of General Psychiatry, 38,* 1293–1295.

Harris, B., Johns, S., Fung, H., Thomas, R., Walker, R., Read, G., & Riad-Fahmy, D. (1989). The hormonal environment of post-natal depression. *British Journal of Psychiatry, 154,* 660–667.

Hays, W.L. (1988). *Statistics* (4th Ed.). Fort Worth, TX: Holt, Rinehart and Winston (pp. 313–315).

Hayworth, J., Little, B.C., Carter, S.B., Raptopoulos, P., Priest, R.G., & Sandler, M. (1980). A predictive study of post-partum depression: Some predisposing characteristics. *British Journal of Medical Psychology, 53,* 161–167.

Henderson, A.F., Gregoire, A.J.P., Kumar, R., & Studd, J.W. (1991). Treatment of severe postnatal depression with oestradiol skin patches. *The Lancet, 338,* 816–817.

Holden, J.M., Sagovsky, R., & Cox, J.L. (1989). Counselling in a general practice setting: Controlled study of health visitor intervention in treatment of postnatal depression. *British Medical Journal, 298,* 223–226.

Hollingshead, A.B. (1975). *Four factor index of social status.* Unpublished manuscript, Yale University, New Haven, CT.

Holmes, T.H., & Rahe, R.H. (1967). The social readjustment rating scale. *Journal of Psychosomatic Research, 11,* 213–218.

Hopkins, J. (1984). *Postpartum depression: The syndrome and its relationship to stress, infant characteristics and social support.* Unpublished doctoral thesis. University of Pittsburgh.

Hopkins, J., Campbell, S.B., & Marcus, M. (1987). The role of infant-related stressors in postpartum depression. *Journal of Abnormal Psychology, 96,* 237–241.

Iles, S., Gath, D., & Kennerley, H. (1989). Maternity blues II. A comparison between post-operative women and post-natal women. *British Journal of Psychiatry, 155,* 363–366.

Jacobson, L., Kaij, L., & Nilsson, A. (1965). Post-partum mental disorders in an unselected sample: Frequency of symptoms and predisposing factors. *British Medical Journal,* 1640–1643.

Jolivet, A., Blanchier, H., & Gautray, J.P. (1974). Blood cortisol variations during late pregnancy and labor. *American Journal of Obstetrics and Gynecology, 119,* 775–783.

Kelsey, J.L., Thompson, W.D., & Evans, A.S. (1986). *Methods in observational epidemiology.* New York: Oxford University Press.

Kendell, R.E. (1985). Emotional and physical factors in the genesis of puerperal mental disorders. *Journal of Psychosomatic Research, 29,* 3–11.

Kendell, R.E., Chalmers, J.C., & Platz, C. (1987). Epidemiology of puerperal psychoses. *British Journal of Psychiatry, 150,* 662–673.

Kendell, R.E., Mackenzie, W.E., West, C., McGuire, R.J., & Cox, J.L. (1984). Day-to-day mood changes after childbirth: Further data. *British Journal of Psychiatry, 145,* 620–625.

Kendell, R.E., McGuire, R.J., Connor, Y., & Cox, J.L. (1981). Mood changes in the first three weeks after childbirth. *Journal of Affective Disorders, 3,* 317–326.

Kennerley, H., & Gath, D. (1986). Maternity blues reassessed. *Psychiatric Developments, 4,* 1–17.

Kennerley, H., & Gath, D. (1989a). Maternity blues I. Detection and measurement by questionnaire. *British Journal of Psychiatry, 155,* 356–362.

Kennerley, H., & Gath, D. (1989b). Maternity blues III. Associations with obstetric, psychological, and psychiatric factors. *British Journal of Psychiatry, 155,* 367–373.

Kenny, D.A. (1987). *Statistics for the social and behavioral sciences* (pp. 299–301). Boston: Little, Brown and Company.

Klein, D.C., Fencil-Morse, E., & Seligman, M.E.P. (1976). Learned helplessness, depression, and the attribution of failure. *Journal of Personality and Social Psychology, 33,* 508–516.

Kleinbaum, D.G., Kupper, L.L., Morgenstern, H. (1982). *Epidemiologic research: Principles and quantitative methods.* Belmont, CA: Lifetime Learning Publications.

Klerman, G.L., Weissman, M.M., Rounsaville, B.J., & Chevron, E.S. (1984). *Interpersonal psychotherapy of depression.* New York: Basic Books.

Kuevi, V., Causon, R., Dixson, A.F., Everard, E.M., Hall, J.M., Hole, D., Whitehead, S.A., Wilson, C.A., & Wise, J.C.M. (1983). Plasma amine and hormone changes in "post-partum blues." *Clinical Endocrinology, 19,* 39–46.

Kumar, R. (1991, October). *Puerperal psychoses: Possibilities for prevention.* Paper presented at the conference on Prevention of Depression After Childbirth: Use and Misuse of the Edinburgh Postnatal Depression Scale, University of Keele, Staffordshire, England.

Kumar, R., & Robson, K.M. (1984). A prospective study of emotional disorders in childbearing women. *British Journal of Psychiatry, 144,* 35–47.

Kupper, L.L., Karon, J.M., Kleinbaum, D.G., Morgenstern, H., Lewis, D.K. (1981). Matching in epidemiologic studies: Validity and efficiency considerations. *Biometrics, 37,* 271–291.

Lanczik, M., Spingler, H., Heidrich, A., Becker, T., Kretzer, B., Albert, P., & Fritze, J. (1992). Postpartum blues: Depressive disease or pseudoneurasthenic syndrome. *Journal of Affective Disorders, 25,* 47–52.

Lazarus, R.S., & Folkman, S. (1984). *Stress, appraisal, and coping.* New York: Springer.

Lee, E. (1980). *Statistical methods for survival analysis.* Belmont, CA: Lifetime Learning Publications.

Lee, E., & Desu, M. (1972). A computer program for comparing *k* samples with right censored data. *Computer Programs in Biomedicine, 2,* 315–321.

Lehman, L. (1985). The relationship of depression to other DSM-III Axis I disorders. In E.E. Beckham & W.R. Leber (Eds.), *Handbook of depression: Treatment, assessment, and research* (pp. 220–315). Homewood, IL: Dorsey.

Levy, V. (1987). The maternity blues in post-partum and post-operative women. *British Journal of Psychiatry, 151,* 368–372.

Lewinsohn, P.M., Hoberman, H.M., & Rosenbaum, M. (1988). A prospective study of risk factors for unipolar depression. *Journal of Abnormal Psychology, 97,* 251–264.

Lewinsohn, P.M., Youngren, M.A., & Grosscup, S.J. (1979). Reinforcement and depression. In R.A. Depue (Ed.), *The psychobiology of depressive disorders: Implications for the effects of stress* (pp. 291–316). New York: Academic Press.

Livingston, J.E., MacLeod, P.M., & Applegarth, D.A. (1978). Vitamin B6 status in women with postpartum depression. *The American Journal of Clinical Nutrition, 31,* 886–891.

Lubin, B. (1965). Adjective check lists for measurement of depression. *Archives of General Psychiatry, 12,* 57–62.

Manly, P.C., McMahon, R.B., Bradley, C.F., & Davidson, P.O. (1982). Depressive attributional style and depression following childbirth. *Journal of Abnormal Psychology, 91,* 245–254.

Mann, J.J., McBride, P.A., Brown, R.P., Linnoila, M., Leon, A.C., DeMeo, M., Mieczkowski, T., Myers, J., & Stanley, M. (1992). Relationship between central and peripheral serotonin indexes in depressed and suicidal psychiatric patients. *Archives of General Psychiatry, 49,* 442–446.

Margolin, G., Michelli, J., & Jacobson, N. (1988). Assessment of marital dysfunction. In M. Hersen & A.S. Bellack (Eds.), *Behavioral assessment: A practical handbook* (2nd ed.), pp. 441–489. New York: Pergamon Press.

Marks, M.N., Wieck, A., Checkley, S.A., & Kumar, R. (1992). Contribution of psychological and social factors to psychotic and non-psychotic relapse after childbirth in women with previous histories of affective disorder. *Journal of Affective Disorders, 29,* 253–264.

Martin, C.J., Brown, G.W., Goldberg, D.P., & Brockington, I.F. (1989). Psychosocial stress and puerperal depression. *Journal of Affective Disorders, 16,* 283–293.

Martin, M.E. (1977). A maternity hospital study of psychiatric illness associated with childbirth. *Irish Journal of Medical Science, 146,* 239–244.

McGrath, E., Keita, G.P., Strickland, B.R., & Russo, N.F. (Eds.) (1990). *Women and depression: Risk factors and treatment issues.* Washington, DC: American Psychological Association.

McNeil, T.F. (1986). A prospective study of postpartum psychoses in a high-risk group. 1. Clinical characteristics of the current postpartum episodes. *Acta Psychiatrica Scandinavica, 74,* 205–216.

Mendlewicz, J. (1985). Genetic research in depressive disorders. In E.E. Beckham & W.R. Leber (Eds.), *Handbook of depression: Treatment, assessment, and research* (pp. 795–815). Homewood, IL: Dorsey.

Metz, A., Cowen, P.J., Gelder, M.G., Stump, K., Elliott, J.M., & Grahame-Smith, D.G. (1983). Changes in platelet $alpha_2$ adrenoceptor binding postpartum: Possible relation to maternity blues. *Lancet, ii,* 495–498.

Monroe, S.M., Bromet, E.J., Connell, M.M., & Steiner, S.C. (1986). Social support, life events, and depressive symptoms: A one-year prospective study. *Journal of Consulting and Clinical Psychology, 54,* 424–431.

Monroe, S.M., & Peterman, A.M. (1988). Life stress and psychopathology. In L.H. Cohen (Ed.), *Life events and psychological functioning: Theoretical and methodological issues* (pp. 31–63). Newbury Park, CA: Sage.

Monroe, S.M., & Simons, A.D. (1991). Diathesis-stress theories in the context of life stress research: Implications for the depressive disorders. *Psychological Bulletin, 110,* 406–425.

Mueller, D.P. (1980). Social networks: A promising direction for research on the relationship of the social environment to psychiatric disorder. *Social Science and Medicine, 14a,* 147–161.

Murray, L. (1992). The impact of postnatal depression on infant development. *Journal of Child Psychology and Psychiatry, 33,* 543–561.

Myers, J.K., Weissman, M.M., Tischler, G.L., Holzer, C.E., Leaf, P.J., Orvaschel, H., Anthony, J.C., Boyd, J.H., Burke, J.D., Jr., Kramer, M., & Stoltzman, R. (1984). Six-month prevalence of psychiatric disorders in three communities. *Archives of General Psychiatry, 41,* 959–967.

Nieland, M.N.S., & Roger, D. (April 1993). *What is postnatal depression?* Paper presented at the annual conference of the British Psychological Society, Blackpool, England.

Nilsson, A., & Almgren, P.E. (1970). Para-natal emotional adjustment: A prospective investigation of 165 women, Part II. *Acta Psychiatrica Scandinavica, Supplementum 220,* 62–141.

Nott, P.N. (1982). Psychiatric illness following childbirth in Southampton: A case register study. *Psychological Medicine, 12,* 557–561.

Nott, P.N. (1987). Extent, timing and persistence of emotional disorders following childbirth. *British Journal of Psychiatry, 151,* 523–527.

Nott, P.N., Franklin, M., Armitage, C., & Gelder, M.G. (1976). Hormonal changes in mood in the puerperium. *British Journal of Psychiatry, 128,* 379–383.

Oakley, A. (1980). *Women confined—towards a sociology of childbirth.* Oxford: Martin Robertson.

O'Hara, M.W. (1986). Social support, life events, and depression during pregnancy and the puerperium. *Archives of General Psychiatry, 43,* 569–573.

O'Hara, M.W. (1987). Post-partum "blues," depression, and psychosis: A review. *Journal of Psychosomatic Obstetrics and Gynaecology, 7,* 205–227.

O'Hara, M.W. (1989). Issues in a controlled study of postpartum depression. In E. van Hall & W. Everaerd (Eds.), *The free woman: Women's health in the 1990's* (pp. 380–387). Carnforth, England: Parthenon Publishing.

O'Hara, M.W. (1991). Postpartum mental disorders. In J.J. Sciarra (Ed.), *Gynecology and Obstetrics,* Vol. 6, Ch. 84. Philadelphia, PA: Harper & Row.

O'Hara, M.W., Neunaber, D.J., & Zekoski, E.M. (1984). A prospective study of postpartum depression: Prevalence, course, and predictive factors. *Journal of Abnormal Psychology, 93,* 158–171.

O'Hara, M.W., & Rehm, L.P. (1979). Self-monitoring, activity levels and mood in the development and maintenance of depression. *Journal of Abnormal Psychology, 88,* 450–453.

O'Hara, M.W., Rehm, L.P., & Campbell, S.B. (1982). Predicting depressive symptomatology: Cognitive-behavioral models and postpartum depression. *Journal of Abnormal Psychology, 91,* 457–461.

O'Hara, M.W., Rehm, L.P., & Campbell, S.B. (1983). Postpartum depression: A role for social network and life stress variables. *Journal of Nervous and Mental Disease, 171,* 336–341.

O'Hara, M.W., Schlechte, J.A., Lewis, D.A., & Varner, M.W. (1991). A controlled prospective study of postpartum mood disorders: Psychological, environmental, and hormonal variables. *Journal of Abnormal Psychology, 100,* 63–73.

O'Hara, M.W., Schlechte, J.A., Lewis, D.A., & Wright, E.J. (1991). Prospective study of postpartum blues: Biologic and psychosocial factors. *Archives of General Psychiatry, 48,* 801–806.

O'Hara, M.W., Varner, M.W., & Johnson, S.R. (1986). Assessing stressful life events associated with childbearing: The Peripartum Events Scale. *Journal of Reproductive and Infant Psychology, 4,* 85–98.

O'Hara, M.W., & Zekoski, E.M. (1988). Postpartum depression: A comprehensive review. In R. Kumar & I.F. Brockington (Eds.), *Motherhood and mental illness 2 Causes and consequences* (pp. 17–63). London: Wright.

O'Hara, M.W., Zekoski, E.M., Philipps, L.H., & Wright, E.J. (1990). A controlled prospective study of postpartum mood disorders: Comparison of childbearing and nonchildbearing women. *Journal of Abnormal Psychology, 99,* 3–15.

Paffenbarger, R.S. (1982). Epidemiological aspects of mental illness associated with childbearing. In I.F. Brockington & R. Kumar (Eds.), *Motherhood and mental illness* (pp. 19–36). New York: Grune & Stratton.

Paykel, E.W. (1979). Recent life events in the development of depressive disorders. In R. Depue (Ed.), *The psychobiology of the depressive disorders* (pp. 245–262). New York: Academic Press.

Paykel, E.S. (1982). Life events and early environment. In E.S. Paykel (Ed.), *Handbook of affective disorders* (pp. 146–161). New York: Guilford Press.

Paykel, E.S., Emms, E.M., Fletcher, J., & Rassaby, E.S. (1980). Life events and social support in puerperal depression. *British Journal of Psychiatry, 136,* 339–346.

Philipps, L.H.C., & O'Hara, M.W. (1991). Prospective study of postpartum depression: 4½-year follow-up of women and children. *Journal of Abnormal Psychology, 100,* 151–155.

Pilkonis, P.A., Imber, S.D., & Rubinsky, P. (1985). Dimensions of life stress in psychiatric patients. *Journal of Human Stress, 11,* 5–10.

Pitt, B. (1968). "Atypical" depression following childbirth. *British Journal of Psychiatry, 114,* 1325–1335.

Pitt, B. (1973). "Maternity blues." *British Journal of Psychiatry, 122,* 431–433.

Playfair, H.R., & Gowers, J.I. (1981). Depression following childbirth—a search for predictive signs. *The Journal of the Royal College of General Practitioners, 31,* 201–208.

Pop, V.J.M., de Rooy, H.A.M., Vader, H.L., van der Heide, D., van Son, M., Komproe, I.H., Essed, G.G.M., & de Geus, C.A. (1991). Postpartum thyroid dysfunction and depression in an unselected population. *New England Journal of Medicine, 324,* 1815–1816.

PSI News: The newsletter for Postpartum Support International (1993). *4,* No. 3, 927 N. Kellogg Avenue, Santa Barbara, CA 93111.

Purdy, D., & Frank, E. (1993). Should postpartum mood disorders be given a more prominent or distinct place in the DSM-IV? *Depression, 1,* 59–70.

Railton, I.E. (1961). The use of corticoids in postpartum depression. *Journal of American Medical Women's Association, 16,* 450–452.

Rehm, L.P. (1977). A self-control model of depression. *Behavior Therapy, 8,* 787–804.

Rehm, L.P. (1988). Assessment of depression. In M. Hersen & A.S. Bellack (Eds.), *Behavioral assessment: A practical handbook* (2nd ed.) (pp. 246–295). New York: Pergamon Press.

Rehm, L.P., Kornblith, S.J., O'Hara, M.W., Lamparski, D.M., Romano, J.M., & Volkin, J. (1981). An evaluation of the major elements in a self-control therapy program for depression. *Behavior Modification, 5,* 459–489.

Robinson, G.E., Olmsted, M.P., & Garner, D.M. (1989). Predictors of postpartum adjustment. *Acta Psychiatrica Scandinavica, 80,* 561–565.

Robinson, G.E., Stewart, D.E., & Flak, E. (1986). The rational use of psychotropic drugs in pregnancy and postpartum. *Canadian Journal of Psychiatry, 31,* 183–190.

Schlesser, M.A. (1986). Neuroendocrine abnormalities in affective disorder. In A.J. Rush & K.Z. Altshuler (Eds.), *Depression: Basic mechanisms, diagnosis, and treatment* (pp. 45–71). New York: Guilford.

Seligman, M.E.P., Abramson, L.Y., Semmel, A., & von Baeyer, C. (1979). Depressive attributional style. *Journal of Abnormal Psychology, 88,* 242–247.

Shapiro, S., Skinner, E.A., Kessler, L.G., von Kroff, M., German, P.S., Tischler, G.L., Leaf, P.J., Benham, L., Cottler, L., & Regier, D.A. (1984). Utilization of health and mental health services. *Archives of General Psychiatry, 41,* 971–982.

Sichel, D.A., Cohen, L.S., Dimmock, J.A., & Rosenbaum, J.F. (1993). Postpartum obsessive-compulsive disorder: A case series. *Journal of Clinical Psychiatry, 54,* 48–51.

Singh, B., Gilhotra, M., Smith, R., Brinsmead, M., Lewin, T., & Hall, C. (1986). Postpartum psychoses and the dexamethasone suppression test. *Journal of Affective Disorders, 11,* 173–177.

Solthau, A., & Taylor, R. (1982). Depression after childbirth. *British Medical Journal, 284,* 980–981.

Spangler, W.D. (1992). Validity of questionnaire and TAT measures of need for achievement: Two meta-analyses. *Psychological Bulletin, 112,* 140–154.

Spanier, G.B. (1976). Measuring dyadic adjustment: New scales for assessing the quality of marriage and similar dyads. *Journal of Marriage and the Family, 38,* 15–28.

Speroff, L., Glass, R.H., & Kase, N.G. (1989). *Clinical gynecologic endocrinology and infertility.* Baltimore, MD: William and Wilkins.

Spitzer, R.L., Endicott, J., & Robins, E. (1978). Research diagnostic criteria: Rationale and reliability. *Archives of General Psychiatry, 36,* 773–782.

Stein, A., Gath, D.H., Bucher, J., Bond, A., Day, A., & Cooper, P.J. (1991). The relationship between post-natal depression and mother-child interaction. *British Journal of Psychiatry, 158,* 46–52.

Stein, G. (1982). The maternity blues. In I.F. Brockington & R. Kumar (Eds.), *Motherhood and mental illness* (pp. 119–154). New York: Grune and Stratton.

Stein, G.S. (1980). The pattern of mental change and body weight change in the first post-partum week. *Journal of Psychosomatic Research, 24,* 165–171.

Stein, G., Marsh, A., & Morton, J. (1981). Mental symptoms, weight changes and electrolyte excretion in the first post partum week. *Journal of Psychosomatic Research, 25,* 395–408.

Stein, G., Milton, F., Bebbington, P., Wood, K., & Coppen, A. (1976). Relationship between mood disturbances and free and total plasma tryptophan in postpartum women. *British Medical Journal, ii,* 457.

Steiner, M. (1979). Psychobiology of mental disorders associated with childbearing. *Acta Psychiatrica Scandinavica, 60,* 449–464.

Stern, G., & Kruckman, L. (1983). Multi-disciplinary perspectives on postpartum depression: An anthropological critique. *Social Science and Medicine, 17,* 1027–1041.

Surtees, P.G., Dean, C., Ingham, J.G., Kreitman, N.B., Miller, P.McC., & Sashidharan, S.P. (1983). Psychiatric disorder in women from an Edinburgh community: Associations with demographic factors. *British Journal of Psychiatry, 142,* 238–246.

Tod, E.D.M. (1964). Puerperal depression: A prospective epidemiological study. *The Lancet, 2,* 1264–1266.

Troutman, B.R., & Cutrona, C.E. (1990). Nonpsychotic postpartum depression among adolescent mothers. *Journal of Abnormal Psychology, 99,* 69–78.

Uddenberg, N. (1974). Reproductive adaptation in mother and daughter. A study of personality development and adaptation to motherhood. *Acta Psychiatrica Scandinavica, Supplementum 254.*

Uddenberg, N., & Englesson, I. (1978). Prognosis of post partum mental disturbance: A prospective study of primiparous women and their $4\frac{1}{2}$-year-old children. *Acta Psychiatrica Scandinavica, 58,* 201–212.

Vemer, H.M., & Rolland, R. (1981). The dynamics of prolactin secretion during the puerperium in women. *Clinical Endocrinology, 15,* 155–163.

Waldron, H., & Routh, D.K. (1981). The effect of the first child on the marital relationship. *Journal of Marriage and the Family, 43,* 785–788.

Watson, D., & Tellegen, A. (1985). Toward a consensual structure of mood. *Psychological Bulletin, 98,* 219–235.

Watson, J.P., Elliott, S.A., Rugg, A.J., & Brough, D.I. (1984). Psychiatric disorder in pregnancy and the first postnatal year. *British Journal of Psychiatry, 144,* 453–462.

Weintraub, S., Neale, J.M., & Liebert, D.E. (1975). Teacher ratings of children vulnerable to schizophrenia. *American Journal of Orthopsychiatry, 45,* 838–845.

Weissman, A.R., & Beck, A.T. (November 1978). *Development and validation of the Dysfunctional Attitude Scale.* Paper presented at the meeting of the Association of Advancement of Behavior Therapy, Chicago.

Weissman, M.M., & Bothwell, S. (1976). Assessment of social adjustment by patient self-report. *Archives of General Psychiatry, 33,* 1111–1115.

Whiffen, V.E. (1988). Vulnerability to postpartum depression: A prospective multivariate study. *Journal of Abnormal Psychology, 97,* 467–474.

Whiffen, V.E., & Gotlib, I.H. (1989). Infants of postpartum depressed mothers: Temperament and cognitive status. *Journal of Abnormal Psychology, 98,* 274–279.

Whiffen, V.E., & Gotlib, I.H. (1993). Comparison of postpartum and nonpostpartum depression: Clinical presentation, psychiatric history, and psychosocial functioning. *Journal of Consulting and Clinical Psychology, 61,* 485–494.

Wolkind, S.N. (1974). Psychological factors and the minor symptoms of pregnancy. *Journal of Psychosomatic Research, 18,* 161–165.

Wolkind, S.N., Coleman, E., & Ghodsian, M. (1980). Continuities in maternal depression. *International Journal of Family Psychiatry, 1,* 167–182.

Wolman, W.-L., Chalmers, B., Hofmeyr, G.J., & Nikodem, V.C. (1993). Postpartum depression and companionship in the clinical birth environment: A randomized, controlled study. *American Journal of Obstetrics and Gynecology, 168,* 1388–1393.

World Health Organization (1978). Mental disorders: Glossary and guide to their classification in accordance with the ninth revision of the *International Classification of Diseases.* Geneva: WHO.

Wrate, R.M., Rooney, A.C., Thomas, P.F., & Cox, J.L. (1985). Postnatal depression and child development: A three-year follow-up study. *British Journal of Psychiatry, 146,* 622-627.

Yalom, I.D., Lunde, D.T., Moos, R.H., & Hamburg, D.A. (1968). "Postpartum blues" syndrome. *Archives of General Psychiatry, 18,* 16–27.

Youngren, M.A., & Lewinsohn, P.M. (1980). The functional relationship between depression and problematic interpersonal behavior. *Journal of Abnormal Psychology, 89,* 333–341.

Zahn-Waxler, C., McKnew, D.H., Cummings, E.M., Davenport, Y.B., & Radke-Yarrow, M. (1984). Problem behaviors and peer interactions of young children with a manic-depressive parent. *American Journal of Psychiatry, 141,* 236–240.

Zajicek, E. (1981). Psychiatric problems during pregnancy. In S. Wolkind & E. Zajicek (Eds.), *Pregnancy: A psychological and social study* (pp. 57–74). London: Academic Press.

Zuckerman, M., & Lubin, B. (1965). *Manual for the Multiple Affective Adjective Check-List.* San Diego, CA: Educational and Industrial Testing Service.

Index

MIX
Papier aus verantwortungsvollen Quellen
Paper from responsible sources
FSC® C105338

If you have any concerns about our products,
you can contact us on
ProductSafety@springernature.com

In case Publisher is established outside the EU,
the EU authorized representative is:
Springer Nature Customer Service Center GmbH
Europaplatz 3, 69115 Heidelberg, Germany

Printed by Libri Plureos GmbH
in Hamburg, Germany